The Most Effective and Responsible Clinical Training Techniques in Medicine

The Most Effective and Responsible Clinical Training Techniques in Medicine

Alternative Types of Learning in Clinical Specialty-Interest Areas of Family-Practice Medicine (Second Edition)

Gary A. DePaul, PhD
Certified Performance Technologist

Author of Nine Practices of 21st Century Leadership: A Guide to Inspiring Creativity, Innovation, and Engagement

ISBN: 1542487870

ISBN-13: 978-1542487870

BISAC: Medical / Education & Training

Library of Congress Control Number: 2017902369

CreateSpace Independent Publishing Platform
North Charleston, SC

Dedication

To James A. Farmer, Jr.

Professor (retired) and my faculty advisor
University of Illinois at Urbana-Champaign

Contents

Preface to the Second Edition

This is the second edition of my 1998 University of Illinois at Ur-bana-Champaign dissertation, *Alternative Types of Learning in Clinical Specialty-Interest Areas of Family-Practice Medicine*. My intent is to make the second edition more relevant and accessible by professionals involved in clinical training in medicine. Here's what's new in the second edition:

Title

I retitled the second edition to attract a broader audience who seek insight or validation about how they provide clinical medical training effectively and responsibly. I kept the original title as a new subtitle to give the context and the research method.

Structure Changes

The standard chapters that you typically find in a dissertation are: introduction, methodology, findings, and discussion. I divided the first traditional chapter into three chapters:

- Chapter 1: Socialization, Family Practice, and Specialty-Interest Areas
- Chapter 2: Specialty-Interest Area Socialization Models
- Chapter 3: Types of Learning and Training Techniques Used in Professions

I kept the remaining three traditional chapters (now chapters 4-6). In addition, I added the following structural parts:

- This preface
- An introduction to the second edition that summarizes key points of my research
- A glossary

I retitled the original abstract to *Introduction to the First Edition.* I moved the reference section to appear after the appendices instead of before the them. I moved the original acknowledgements to appear after the references.

After the appendices, I replaced the cv with a section entitled, *About the Author.*

Content Changes

As with many manuscripts, authors find mistakes in the text. I corrected these instances. I also updated some concept descriptions. Where I provide stories to illustrate a concept, I included fictional names. For example, instead of referring to "a female FP specialist," I referred the specialist as a name such as "Susan."

To improve readability and to specifically to remove unnecessary complexities, I made several format changes:

- For the headings, I made some minor changes to the titles and improved the heading format.
- I changed the font from Times New Roman to Arial, changed double-spacing to single-spacing, and changed to traditional full justification.
- I made voice changes and used informality to improve readability. As much as possible, I change passive voice to active voice. Instead of referring to myself as *the researcher,* I changed third person to first person. I also added some verb contractions.
- In the first edition, I often lumped *procedures* with *routines,* *protocols,* and *principles.* Where the context made sense, I only used *procedures* to improve readability. For purposes of the second edition, I assume that procedures are rou-

tines, include protocols and policies, and are based on underlying principles. I acknowledge that you can reference routines, protocols, policies, and principle independent of any procedures.

- I converted lists appearing in paragraphs to bullet lists.
- When I emphasized words, I replaced underlined words with italic words.
- I didn't update the references to the current APA style. I did, however, replace underlines with italics. Also, I moved the references to appear after the appendices instead of before them.
- I changed the appendices from letters to roman numerals.
- For key points that I wanted to emphasize, such as the main research question, I indented the left and right sides to create a callout (similar to quotations).
- I recreated the figures and tables and corrected errors from the first edition caused during the microfilm conversion.

Introduction to the Second Edition

*My generation was never explicitly taught
how to think as clinicians. We learned medicine catch-as-catch-can. Trainees observed
senior physicians the way apprentices observed master craftsmen in a medieval
guild, and somehow the novices were sup-
posed to assimilate their elder's approach to
diagnosis and treatment. Rarely did an attending physician actually explain the mental steps that led him to his decisions.*
(4-5)

— Jerome Groopman, MD
How Doctors Think

If you believe the broad aim of clinical training is about teaching
medical procedures, you're wrong. Whether you an attending, a faculty member, or another type of clinical instructor, believing this can
limit or even hinder the learning process.

Granted, a large part of clinical training involves instructing medical procedures. But this isn't enough for preparing professionals for
practicing as specialists or subspecialists. To introduce my research at Carle Clinic Association, I present a broader context on
clinical medical training and some of the research insights from social-cognitive learning. I divide the introduction into five themes and
provide references at the end of this introduction.

Since UMI published the first edition nearly twenty years ago,
I've experienced these five themes while working in various organizations. Although these organizations aren't associated with the

medical field, the themes span across several industries—industries with professionals who argue that their training context is unique. Despite context uniqueness, these themes seem to be universal to several cadre of professionals.

For the rest of this introduction, I discuss each theme:

1. Training doesn't necessarily result in learning.
2. During the training experience, learners can develop unfavorable beliefs and habits.
3. Learning doesn't necessarily transfer to performance (that is, transfer into appropriate behaviors that lead to desirable results).
4. The broad aim of clinical training is to socialize new specialists to the culture of expert practice.
5. Too often, content experts in an instructor's role believe that clinical training isn't complicated and they don't need much preparation, if any.

Theme One: Training Doesn't Necessarily Result in Learning

People learn a wide range of tasks. They learn habits, both good and bad. They learn skills such as operating a forklift or a smartphone. They learn theories, beliefs, and even emotions. Sometimes learning is deliberate while other times it's unconscious.

Learning involves a change in behavior, but it is more than that. Merriam-et al. (2007) define learning this way:

> Learning is a process that brings together cognitive, emotional, and environmental influences and experiences for acquiring, enhancing, or making changes in one's knowledge, skills, values, and worldviews. (277)

Larkin (1989) reminds us that while incidental learning can occur with any experience, not all experiences have intentional learning goals. Larkin uses the label *intentional learning* to refer to cognitive activities that have learning as the goal.

Clinical training has a unique instructional system. Medical facilities tend to pay learners as employees who work under the auspices of a clinical expert. The clinical expert happens to be their instructor. At times, it's unclear when the new professionals function as employees and when as learners. Consider Dr. Samantha Jones, a cardiologist attending. Dr. Jones manages the quality care of patients and the instruction of residents. Often, Dr. Jones focuses exclusively on a patient's presenting problem but leaves residents to figure out on their own what they learn by observing how she works with the patient. At other times, Dr. Jones critiques the residents' knowledge and observations to make explicit what the residents should learn from a specific case.

Residents may fail to appropriately learn due to a lack of information. They may not even reflect upon one of Dr. Jones's cases from a learning perspective. As expressed in the opening quotation of this introduction, learning habitually is *catch-as-catch-can*.

The Instructor's Dilemma

In this book, I discuss various clinical dilemmas. One dilemma I don't discuss is the instructor's dilemma. Instructors struggle with two competing directives: focus on quality patient care and focus on quality instruction.

When instructors emphasize quality patient care and deemphasize instruction, they treat learners as employees who assist instructors with patient care. Instructors give minimal training and may unconsciously expect learners to figure out on their own the cognitive processes and mind-set needed to become experts. If learners can't figure this out, then some instructors might conclude that the learners picked the wrong specialty and shouldn't become this type of clinical specialist.

Sadly, the other extreme of this dilemma happens as well. James A. Farmer Jr., an educational consultant to the American Academy of Orthopaedic Surgery (AAOS) and my graduate-school mentor, shared with me a story about Dr. Johnson (not his real name), an orthopaedic attending. Dr. Johnson wanted to humble Dr. Omar, a brilliant but overconfident and arrogant resident. He told the resident to lead a surgical procedure. While the resident hadn't practiced this particular procedure before, he had assisted Dr. Johnson once. Dr. Johnson knew that the resident would encounter a complication, but he allowed Dr. Omar to proceed without warning. When the procedure went wrong and caused damage to the patient, Dr. Johnson took over, scolded Dr. Omar for his technical incompetence, and then showed the resident what he should have done. Even though the resident learned from the experience, Dr. Johnson did this at the expense of the patient's health. Farmer calls unethical lessons like this one *guided shaming*.

Resolving the instructor's dilemma requires doing both extremes. Quality patient care must be primary, or what I call the *syntonic* choice of a dilemma, and quality instruction must be secondary, or what I call the *dystonic*. To do both effectively, instructors need to be trained on effective instructional techniques and continuously develop their instructional capabilities. Doing so not only improves the quality of instruction for learners, but instructors will inadvertently discover that they become better at providing quality care for their patients.

The Instructor's Mindset

Effective instructors have the mindset of an expert clinical specialist and the instructor's mindset. Part of the instructor's mindset is to consider every clinical experience as an opportunity for learners to develop new knowledge or to practice a procedure or skillset. For Nesher (1989), all instruction is "goal-directed, intentional, and conscious activity and therefore amendable to rational analysis and critical consideration" (187). Instructors accomplish learning goals by guiding, shaping, and supporting novice learning until the instructor's efforts are no longer needed (Brown and Palincsar, 1989). The more accomplished instructors are at effective instruction, the more likely learners will successfully accomplish their clinical training.

Instructors need to recognize that when learners begin a clinical training program, they don't start as empty vessels: their experiences and speculation contribute to preconceived and naive understanding about what the clinical specialist's mindset is. Resnick (1989) summarizes this succinctly:

> People do not come as empty vessels to
> learning. In almost any domain, even beginners carry with them ideas of how things
> work and frameworks for interpreting new

> information...People are sometimes una-
> ware of having them but, nevertheless, use
> them as framework for interpreting situa-
> tions and acting in them. (5)

For example, while I'm not a sports-medicine expert, I have a naive sense of what's involved in providing patient care for sport injuries. If I want to become a sports-medicine specialist, I'd have to either give up or change my naive beliefs.

Instructors need to be aware of where learners are developmentally (in becoming a type of specialist) and anticipate misconceptions that they could have about the clinical specialty and what they need to develop to become a clinical expert.

In "On the Nature of Competence," Gelman and Greeno (1989) describe Glaser's three components needed for a theory of instruction. Before working with learners, clinical instructors need a theory about:

- The knowledge, skills, and mindset needed for learners to become clinical specialists
- The knowledge, skills, and mindset that learners have when starting clinical training
- The instructional process and techniques needed to transition learners from their initial state to the desired state of clinical specialty expertise

The third bullet point includes having instructors consider the instructional environment and related constraints that affect how learners develop their specialty expertise.

Theme Two: During the Training Experience, Learners Can Develop Unfavorable Beliefs and Habits

Instructors responsibly guide learners to give up their naive beliefs and socialize them to what Collins, Brown, and Newman (1989) call a *culture of expert practice* in which expertise is "...the practice of solving problems and carrying out tasks in a domain" (488).

Regrettably, many instructors use ineffective techniques to develop learner expertise. Recall Groopman's quotation at the beginning of this introduction. When instructors model expertise without articulating the cognitive process underlying the behaviors, they leave the explanation to the learners; learners are then forced to derive the cognitive process, often using trial-and-error guesswork. Chi and Bassok (1989) describe requiring learners to construct explanations as incomplete instruction:

> We reasoned that because example-exercises, as we have analyzed, are so incomplete in providing explanations for the action sequences, the students must necessarily construct their own explanations for the sequence of actions in order to understand the materials. (269)

While Chi and Bassok's reasoning is based on a nonclinical environment, Collins, Brown, and Newman (1989) describe this type of instructional inadequacy in a way that applies to a clinical environment:

> However, a learning environment in which experts simply solve problems and carry out tasks, and learners simply watch, is inadequate to provide effective models for learning, particularly in cognitive domains where many of the relevant processes they engage in as they solve problems. (488)

Learners can't explain to themselves with certainty the instructor's complex cognitive process by observation alone. Without having instructors articulate out-loud explanations for what they are doing, learners would have serious challenges in figuring out the cognitive processes behind actions, such as why instructors do the following:

- Ask patients certain questions
- Touch a patient's back before making an incision
- Order unexpected diagnostic tests
- Perform a surgical procedure easily with one patient but with difficulty with another patient

Without explicit instructor explanations, learners are unlikely to perceive behavioral meaning—especially tacit knowledge—such as:

- Underlying principles
- Pattern recognition types
- Heuristics
- Risk management and pitfall avoidance
- Metacognition tactics

Learners guessing what the instructors' cognitive thinking was can be faulty at best and at worst can cause learners to make technical errors that result in patient harm.

Chi and Bassock (1989) argue that instructors need to shape learner explanations. Instructors accomplish this by articulating their thinking aloud during or after an event. For more advanced learners who should have familiarity with such explanations, instructors can ensure that they grasp fully the underlying thinking by asking them questions about the instructor's actions such as the following:

- Why do you think I asked those questions to the patient? What was I wanting to know?
- What conditions would you need before taking that action?
- If you notice this problem occurring when performing this procedure, what should you do?
- What are the principles related to this step?
- What's the worst that could go wrong with this type of patient-treatment plan?
- Even though we diagnosed the symptoms to be caused by this problem, what else could the problem be?
- Under what circumstances would you need to refer the patient with these symptoms to another specialist?
- After performing this procedure, what could have gone wrong? What complications should we watch for?

When instructors give explanations for what learners observe or when they question learners to clarify their understanding, learners can develop the needed cognitive capacities from only a few cases.

With student problem solving, Chi and Bassock (1989) discovered learning can occur from experiencing a small number of examples coupled with explanation:

> ...our data suggest that students can learn, with understanding, from single or a few examples, contrary to the other available empirical evidence...However, only those students who provide adequate explanations during studying are able to see the degree to which they can generalize their problem-solving skills. (280)

Clinical instructors need to model not only the consensually validated behaviors of the specialty; they need to communicate the underlying cognitive processes, especially the tacit knowledge. As learners become more experienced, instructors should focus on validating learner understanding by having learners articulate aloud what they are thinking during or after they perform the behavior. Using questioning, instructors should decide if learners grasp the underlying principles and are capable of generalizing to other relevant situations.

Theme Three: Learning Doesn't Necessarily Transfer to Performance

In *Performance-Focused Smile Sheets*, Will Thalheimer discusses two important training concepts: the *learning* curve and the *forgetting* curve. As novice professionals' learning increases over time, they simultaneously forget knowledge as well. After completing their training, their learning continues but so does their forgetting. What's forgotten can't transfer to performance, and just because new specialists learn something doesn't mean that they will apply that knowledge in medical practice.

Clinical instructors can choose one of two paths. On the first path, they don't help learners figure out how to retain knowledge, skills, and the clinical mindset. On the second path, instructors assume more responsibility and help learners with retention and, consequently, improve future performance.

Knowing Resnick's (1989) perspective on the function of instruction can help clinical instructors more effectively assist learners. As

Resnick notes, learners have a difficult time retaining isolated facts, including rote memorization. Simply memorizing knowledge alone is not learning. Instead, learners can effectively retain facts if they do two things.

First, learners should interpret facts so that the knowledge is meaningful to them. Brown and Palincsar (1989) call this *internalization* and *personalization*: learners articulate the knowledge using their own words but within the profession's constraints. Internalization may occur later in the learning process, such as after getting a certain amount of practice applying the knowledge.

Second, retention can be more effective when learners embed the knowledge in some type of organizing structure for future retrieval—sometimes called *mental models*. The better learners are at building relational connections among different sets of knowledge, the better the retention.

Clinical-instructional theory should involve more than communicating knowledge and allowing learners enough practice applying techniques; it should strive to enable learners to construct mental models. Like a web, knowledge needs to connect with other knowledge, forming an elaborate, interconnecting cognitive system. This system approximates what learners should know about their role in the profession's specialty.

Too often, content experts in an instructor's role believe that clinical training isn't complicated and doesn't require much preparation, if any. Effective clinical training is not easy. Resnick (1989) describes instruction as a type of intervention:

> Instruction must provide information for learners' knowledge construction process. It must constrain those processes so that they will result in knowledge that is both true and powerful... (2)

If instruction is a type of intervention that stimulates learners to construct mental models of their specialization, learners could benefit by knowing this. Instructors guide and encourage learners to connect and generalize principles and beliefs to different contexts; this can strengthen the learning process, decrease some of the forgetting, and increase learning transfer to performance.

Clinical instructors can help learners organize new knowledge.

They can explain and reinforce how principles and techniques can apply to different situations and when using the techniques types of situations would be contraindicated. Navigating learners through such complexities can strengthen their mental model and help them avoid technical errors.

Theme Four: The Broad Aim of Clinical Training Is to Socialize New Specialists to the Culture of Expert Practice

The first night of internship showed me that I needed to think differently from how I had learned to think in medical school... (33)

—Jerome Groopman, MD
How Doctors Think

Even though learning diagnostics and therapeutic treatment procedures is necessary to develop expertise in a specialty, it isn't enough. Beyond developing procedural expertise, new professionals need to learn how their roles think and function within a clinical setting. Hence, they need to learn the culture of expert practice.

Collins et al. (1989) describe a *culture of expert practice* as a learning environment in which professionals communicate and engage in activities at an expertise level. While learning from expert specialists, both novice and expert share in problem solving. By doing so, learners become sensitized to the details of expert performance and adjust their performance to approximate expertise performance. Collins et al. state:

A culture of expert practice helps situate and support learning [for novices]...a culture focused on expert practice provides learners with the readily available models of expert-in-use; as we discussed, the availability of such models helps learners build and refine a conceptual model of the tasks they are trying to carry out. (488)

As I quoted earlier, Collins et al. warn that having learners only watch experts work isn't enough to develop expertise:

> However, a learning environment in which
> experts simply solve problems and carry out
> tasks, and learners simply watch, is inade-
> quate to provide effective models for learn-
> ing, particularly in cognitive domains where
> many of the relevant processes they en-
> gage in as they solve problems. Drawing
> students into a culture of expert practice in
> cognitive domains involves teaching them
> how to "think like experts." (488)

The key for successfully becoming a specialist involves having new professionals learn how to *think like experts* and develop their capability to adapt to the culture as it relates to their role. In *Helping People Win at Work*, Blanchard and Ridge (2009) define culture in the following way:

> ...the assumptions, beliefs, values, cus-
> toms, and behaviors of the organization's
> employees, supervisors, and leaders. In
> other words, culture is "the way we do
> things around here." (43)

To adapt to a culture, especially one that requires expert practice (and anything less than expertise is unacceptable for patient care), new professionals must learn and internalize a great deal that isn't clear through observation. They must learn the cognition underlying observable behaviors. In figure i, I illustrate the subtle aspects of culture with an iceberg analogy. Above the water surface is the tip of the iceberg. The tip symbolizes all the behaviors of their new role that is more readily observable and easier for them to socialize and adapt to, including some of the cognitive processes that are more explicit, such as the following:

• The clinical setting
• Patients presenting health problems
• Procedural training
• Well-known constraints such as the Hippocratic Oath
• Training performance feedback

Physical environment including building
layout, equipment, supplies, patient charts,
uniforms, background sounds, signage,
posted branding such as values and mission
statement, medical and nonmedical
personnel, patients, and patient visitors

Presenting problems
and symptoms

Potential procedural difficulties due to blameless errors,
blameworthy errors, inevitable complications, constructive
and destructive bugs, and untoward events

Leverage heuristics
and tricks-of-the-trade

The Specialist's

Minimize emotions, biases,
influences, and dilemmas (as much
as reasonably possible)

Rescue and

Codified rescue: whole and fragmented
procedures (includes compromised
rescue)

Training

For expert specialists encountering
unknown territory: referral or individual
innovation

Others

Socializing learners to
behaviors and cognitive
mindset of the profession

Learning how to instruct clinical procedures
to new specialists effectively and responsibly

Figure i. Learning a Clinical Specialty Iceberg Model

Explicit constraints imposed by laws, organization's administration, the medical profession (Hippocratic Oath), and the medical specialty

Learning and performance feedback and evaluations

Diagnostic and therapeutic procedures development

For each procedure: underlying principles, cognitive thinking on how to execute the steps, knowledge about potential complications, errors, and how to handle or avoid them

Mindset

Shared values, beliefs, ethical codes specific to the specialty, power structure, cultural and relationship norms, and idiosyncrasies/personalization

Recovery

Address housestaff normative and quasi-normative errors

Training

Others

Acknowledge errors (self-discipline) such as through morbidity and mortality (M&M) conferences

Manage and monitor learner development

Mitigate and minimize learners' buggy thinking

In the illustration, the area just at the water level and the first part of the submerged iceberg symbolizes the cognitive processes and learners' reasonably deduced explanations for expert behaviors. Part of this includes learner recognition that diagnostic and therapeutic treatment procedures have an element of the unknown and can cause unexpected but often manageable complications. Clues to the causes are somewhat clear at this level. Causes include professional errors and nonstandard patient conditions.

Deeper below the surface is the hidden and larger part of the iceberg. Here, the water is murky and symbolizes how much of cognitive knowledge is not apparent through observation alone, and even experts who instruct have difficulty articulating to learners their tacit knowledge. How do attendings, for example, articulate to learners how, in the matter of seconds, they can diagnose a patient's condition by using pattern recognition fueled by decades of experience?

I characterize the hidden bulk of the iceberg as three levels:

- The specialist's mindset
- Rescue and recovery
- Training others

I describe each in the rest of this section.

The Specialist's Mindset

Relationship Norms

A critical aspect of a culture of expert practice involves how the role interacts with other roles. New professionals need to learn, for example, how experts talk with patients, how much of their diagnoses and treatment they explain, what they should withhold from patients, and the ethical consequences of withholding information, including the specialist's opinions. They need to consider questions such as:

- Is it in the patient's best interest to share concerns, even though the concerns might not materialize, or should the specialist wait until the concerns are realized?
- How would sharing concerns positively or negatively affect the patient?

How a specialist interacts with others involves a range of conditions. These need to be taken seriously and with great respect. New specialists must develop how they interact appropriately with other roles, including

- Administrators
- Attorneys and external auditors
- Colleagues within the same specialty and other types of specialists
- Housestaff
- Law enforcement
- Patient relations
- Patients
- Pharmaceutical and device representatives
- Residents, interns, and medical students

Forgive and Remember: Clinical Errors

In his book *Forgive and Remember*, Bosk (2003) immersed himself among surgeons in his ethnographical study at a teaching hospital. Bosk discovered that, beyond instructing diagnosis and treatment, the faculty instructs professional self-control to avoid and decrease errors. Bosk identified two error categories: *blameless* and *blameworthy.*

Bosk describes blameless errors as technical and judgmental. Both are an inevitable part of practice for anyone. When specialists recognize these errors, they admit them and seek to rectify and learn from the experience.

> Technical offenses are forgiven by superordinates. This leniency promotes cohesion among members of the work force. Forgiveness itself operates as a deterrence to further technical error. First, it obligates the subordinate who is forgiven to the superordinate who shows him mercy. To repay this obligation, the subordinate becomes more vigilant in the immediate future…Second, when a subordinate sees his technical errors are forgiven, he recognizes that he has

> no incentive to hide them. He is less likely,
> therefore, to compound his problems by at-
> tempting to treat problems that are over his
> head for fear of superordinate reprisal. For-
> giveness encourages "help-seeking" behav-
> ior and removes the stigma from uncer-
> tainty.
>
> Forgiveness also serves to reintegrate of-
> fenders into the group...
>
> ...forgiveness serves to limit self-criticism
> and prevent an individual from being immo-
> bilized by guilt. Forgiveness helps individu-
> als mobilize for action after failure has
> stripped them of a sense of mastery.
> (178–79)

Unless technical and judgmental errors are repeated, learners are forgiven, and the faculty permits learners to complete their training.

Bosk labels the more severe and blameworthy errors as norma-tive and quasi-normative. Because medicine isn't perfect, honest errors are inevitable. Nevertheless, the cadre of professionals ex-pects perfect compliance to ethical norms:

> ...physicians do expect perfect compliance
> with the norms of clinical responsibil-
> ity...Negligence is defined in terms of clini-
> cal norms—moral values—and not technical
> standards. (181)

Normative errors are violations of standards held by the special-ists. When these occur, Bosk notes that the superordinates view these as severe and intolerant, and in the short run, this leads to shaming and punishment along with pressure for learners to prove that the error is a rare exception:

> The onus then falls on the subordinate to
> show that his lapse was only temporary and
> not representative of his work. He must
> show that he "has learned his lesson and
> been properly put in his place." Those who

> cannot demonstrate this in the long run are
> excommunicated from the group... (179)

Bosk illustrates a normative error by describing a resident who fought with the nursing staff. The standard is that the faculty expects specialists who have better training and are "supposedly more mature than staff" (56) to get along with the nursing staff. Not doing so, regardless of what the staff has done to warrant the ire of the specialist, is unacceptable.

The other blameworthy error is more curious and can potentially interfere with the learning process. Quasi-normative errors are violations of the instructor's idiosyncrasies and style:

> ...attending A and attending B view the differences between themselves as nothing more than an artifact of training, clinical experience, individual philosophy, personality—in a word, as a difference in style. In this setting, differences of style among colleagues are recognized as legitimate... Quasi-normative errors—that is, the stylistic idiosyncrasies of attendings—serve to isolate the surgical services from one another.
> ...quasi-normative error serves as a device to maintain the boundary between attending and housestaff. (186)

Quasi-normative errors are not agreed upon by the cadre of professionals, so these errors are violations of an instructor's worldview. Learners have the challenge to discover each instructor's boundaries and act in ways to avoid making quasi-normative errors.

> Quasi-normative errors are eccentric and attending-specific. Each attending has certain protocols that he [sic] and he [sic] alone follows. A subordinate who does not follow these rules mocks his superordinate's authority. (227)

Instructors punish and shame learners for quasi-normative errors in the same way as normative errors. Bosk finds this problematic. Because instructors treat quasi-normative errors like normative ones, learners can have difficulty deciding what is normative and what isn't. When one instructor perceives an act as a violation, learners may mistakenly believe a quasi-normative error to be normative. Worse, learners could mistakenly assume a normative error as being quasi-normative and believe that another instructor wouldn't consider the act to be an error.

During clinical training, instructors should explicitly discuss the profession's expectations about errors and clarify how learners should rectify the situation when they make errors. I'm not implying that instructors should do this formally like a classroom, but they should informally discuss error expectations and give examples often. The more open instructors are about tacit aspects of the culture, the more likely learners will adapt appropriately.

Heuristics

Scarlett (2016) states that our brains like shortcuts that save us time and effort. Specialists have shortcuts that they often referred to as *heuristics* and *tricks-of-the*-trade. With the multiple decisions specialists make daily, these can help specialists reserve energy and more effectively work with patients over their long hours.

Scarlett (2016) warns, though, that shortcuts can be dangerous and cause flawed decision making. When we view the world through our shortcuts, we see clinical problems from a distorted view. Instructors need to train learners on these shortcuts as well as on their limitations.

Cognitive Biases and External Influence

> *The brain is designed with blind spots, optical and psychological, and one of its cleverest tricks is to confer on us the comforting delusion that we, personally, do not have any.* (42)

> —Carol Travis and Elliot Aronson
> *Mistakes Were Made (But Not by Me)*

In corporate training and leadership development, there's been an increased interest in the effect of cognitive bias on how teams work and on organizational change. Recent books, such as Scarlett's 2016 *Neuroscience for Organizational Change*, explain how training on these biases can improve performance. Similarly, in his 2008 book, *How Doctors Think*, Groopman describes cognitive biases that influence the specialist's decisions and explains how training on them can help decrease their negative effect. He specifically discusses representative bias, attribution errors, affective errors, confirmation bias, anchoring, commission bias, and satisfaction-of-search bias (to name a few). In addition to these biases, Groopman explains how pharmaceutical representatives can influence prescription behaviors and how insurance payment policies to doctors can influence the types of procedures used—even when the procedure isn't in the patient's best interest. Groopman, though, carefully explains that doctors may be unaware of these influences.

Along with instructing cognitive processes and tacit knowledge, instructors need to help new professionals learn about these biases and share tactics to minimize their negative influence.

Clinical Dilemmas

A critical finding in my research has to do with the dilemmas that family-practice specialists must address when developing specialty-interest areas. In chapters 5 and 6, I describe a three-way interlocking dilemma consisting of these dilemmas:

- Autonomy vs. control
- Procedures vs. invention
- Safe practice vs. risky practice

Dilemmas have two opposing viewpoints that can be attractive to specialists. Either can benefit specialists, but in some circumstances, they can also cause harm. The dilemma resolution is to accept both but consider one as the primary and the other as secondary. I label these as syntonic and dystonic. For example, with the procedure vs. invention dilemma, specialists need to learn the circumstances in which they need to follow consensually validated procedures and the circumstances when inventing solutions is indicated.

Bosk (2003) and Groopman (2008) identify additional dilemmas that instructors should discussed explicitly as part of clinical training.

Cost-containment vs. liability management

With patient-case management, specialists grapple between doing too much or too little. At one extreme, insurance companies, the government, and sometimes patients pressure specialists to perform the minimal services necessary to resolve patient health problems. At the other extreme, if specialists fail to resolve patient problems because they didn't do enough, patients could experience serious and harmful consequences, and specialists could be liable. Instructors need to model and clarify the conditions to learners that help them navigate between these two extremes.

Detachment/suppressed emotions vs. caring/concern

Groopman (2008) eloquently explains this dilemma:

> If we feel our emotions deeply, we risk recoiling or breaking down. If we erase our emotions, however, we fail to care for the patient. We face a paradox: feeling prevents us from being blind to our patient's soul but risks blinding us to what is wrong with him. (54)

Moreover, caring too much or not enough can bias specialists and interfere with doing what's best for helping and treating patients.

As with any dilemma, instructors need to help learners navigate a balance between the two extremes—in this case, detachment and caring. Some could argue that this needs to be experienced first-hand and self-taught, but instructors can expedite the learning process and potentially prevent any major developmental setbacks.

Limited questioning vs lengthy questioning

Groopman (2008) warns that the questions specialists ask shape and bias patient response. If specialists gather a history too quickly, they could form the wrong diagnosis. If, however, they delve too deeply, this takes time from other patients and interferes with other duties. Instructors need to model asking the type of questions that have been consensually validated by the profession. They need to help learners comprehend the rationale for these questions, and they need to enable learners to obtain the appropriate history needed to help patients with their health problems.

Zebra Dilemma

Groopman (2008) introduces Pat Croskerry's term *zebra retreat* when deciding a diagnosis. He writes:

> Another echoing maxim on rounds: "When you hear hoofbeats, think about horses, not zebras." (126)

For Croskerry, *zebra retreat* occurs when specialists avoid making rarely occurring diagnosis. Groopman links this dilemma with the cost containment vs. liability management dilemma:

> Powerful forces in modern medicine discourage hunting for them...In an era of cost containment, when insurers and managed care plans scrutinize how much physicians spend on any one patient, doctors have a strong disincentive to pursue ideas that are "out there." (126)

Statistically, patient's presenting problems would fall into the more common category, but unfortunately, some patients go years without problem resolution when specialists see horses rather than zebras. From personal empiricism, I've seen this happening, and the result of not diagnosing the rare condition left one patient partially blind and another with brain damage.

Groopman explains that instructors need to train residents to keep in mind the critical question: "What's the worst explanation for this condition?" Modeling this question should help train specialists keep an open mind for other possibilities.

Rescue and Recovery

In the iceberg model, at the rescue-and-recovery level, I list codified rescue and unknown territory, and I describe in chapter 6.

As part of clinical training, instructors need to train learners on how to rescue and recover from errors and unforeseen complications. Some rescue procedures are well defined while others are fragmented—a type of heuristic. In extreme situations, specialists cannot recover without some cost to patients. These are compromised rescues that involve whole or fragmented procedures.

Also at this level, I list addressing errors. Instructors should prepare learners to acknowledge their errors and set expectations for addressing them—regardless if handled informally or through a formal channel such as morbidity and mortality (M&M) conferences. What's critical is for learners to adapt to a culture of atonement and learn from their errors to become better healers.

Training Others

From a social-cognitive learning perspective[1], effective clinical instruction involves making tacit knowledge—principles, beliefs, and cognitive processes—explicit within the context. Learning the behaviors of procedural steps without explanation isn't acceptable or responsible. Also irresponsible are instructional techniques that promote discovery or trial-and-error learning in a clinical setting that requires expert practice to provide the highest care for patients.

To be clear, the techniques I describe in these chapters are all legitimate (except for guided shaming). However, some are more suitable for clinical training, and the context indicates which techniques are the most effective, responsible, and applicable. Learning techniques used in primary and secondary education that promote experimentation and self-discovery are applaudable. Yet these techniques would be inappropriate for clinical training that relies on consensually validated standards of practice, constraints for protecting patient health, and dire consequences if new professionals are encourage to deviate from the standards. In the chapter 3, I describe these learning techniques:

- Autonomous learning
- Cognitive apprenticeship and BOGERD
- Guided inquiry

- Reception learning
- Socratic learning

Rather than repeat what I wrote about the techniques in chapter 3 and appendix I, note that, given the specific context, these techniques are appropriate in clinical training, except for guided inquiry. The following are examples for using the learning techniques.

- *Cognitive Apprenticeship*: This learning technique is most effective for instructing expert practice of complex tasks in which the related cognitive process is more critical to learn than just the behavioral movements. Collins et al. (1989) explain that the technique is designed to bring tacit processes into the open by having learners start by observing instructors and later by practicing the procedures with help from instructors and even more experienced learners.
- Socratic Learning: After learners have exposure to knowledge (for example, after the first two phases of cognitive apprenticeship), instructors can use this technique to encourage learners to elaborate their comprehension and to test the boundaries or applicability of that knowledge. Brown and Palincsar (1989) explain that instructors can do this using discussion ploys such as:
  - Ask learners about case variations and what they would do differently.
  - Question learner conclusions and faulty reasoning with counterexamples and hypothetical cases.
- *Reception Learning*: Learners can strengthen and fine-tune their mental models by attending conferences, reading journals, and listening to lectures. While this technique is contraindicated for learning a new procedure that is dissimilar to other learned procedures, reception learning can be a powerful learning technique.
- Autonomous Learning: Like reception learning, learners can choose to read journals and medical references on their own to supplement and strengthen their diagnostic and treatment capabilities. So long as the self-directed learning is within the gold standards and supplements (but doesn't replace) social-cognitive learning, this technique can be effective and responsible.

Part of training involves monitoring and managing learner development and ensuring that learners have the necessary exposure and developed capabilities for them to proceed beyond clinical training. Instructors need to take an active role in managing the learner experience rather than just giving the clinical exposure.

Theme Five: Too Often, Content Experts in an Instructor's Role Believe That Clinical Training Isn't Complicated and They Don't Need Much Preparation, If Any

Is it possible to become a clinical instructor without having formal training on clinical instruction? Of course! New instructors can reflect upon how instructors trained them and then try to approximate the perceived instructional behaviors.

For example, Dr. Jones, a new attending cardiologist, did just that. In his role, he diagnoses and treats patients while allowing residents to observe, and he occasionally explains to residents his reasoning for actions taken. Dr. Jones leaves some of the simpler procedures to the residents, questions residents during rounds, and supports them when they are on call. Occasionally, though, Dr. Jones would make instructional mistakes, but he openly admits his errors and learns from them.

Developing Instructional Capabilities: Two Approaches

Perhaps developing instructional capabilities through trial-and-error learning is the typical approach and is effective to some degree. However, those who are appropriately trained as clinical instructors, study social-cognitive learning theory, and have a clear understanding of the intent of clinical training have a stronger effect on learner development than those who developed their instructional capabilities using trial-and-error learning. Continuously and deliberately developing instructional capabilities increases effectiveness of learner development.

Those who develop their instructional capabilities through trial-and-error learning place most of the responsibility for learning a specialty on learners. Thus, learners either figure out what they need to know and do, or the faculty won't allow them to graduate and be part of the cadre of professionals. In contrast, those who are trained appropriately take a more active role and responsibility for ensuring learners achieve their long-term goals. When learners don't achieve their goals, this reflects poorly on both the instructors and learners. The excuse that learners who fail lacked the needed qualities to succeed, therefore reflecting poorly on the learners alone, isn't acceptable.

There is a moral responsibility for instructors to strengthen their instructional capabilities so that they can effectively enable learners to mature and develop the specialist's mindset and acceptable level of expertise. Wanting their learners to succeed should be enough to motivate continuous development of their instructional capabilities.

Linkage between Leadership and Clinical Instruction

From my research on leadership practices, I discovered a strong linkage between the clinical instructor's role and contemporary leadership. In contrast to traditional leadership or the art of getting things done through others, contemporary leadership is about influencing others to build their character. In other words, leadership is helping those around you to mature their mental and moral qualities, capabilities, and behaviors. As I noted earlier in this introduction, clinical training in a medical specialty or subspecialty is a type of ethical training that increases the learners' capacity to manage a proper level of self-control while diagnosing and treating patients. Thus, a substantial aspect of the clinical instructor's role involves practicing leadership. The more an instructor deliberately assists learners in their development of moral behaviors within the context of the specialty, the more the instructor practices genuine leadership.

Learning instructional practices by trial and error has a narrow perspective of the purpose of clinical training: such instructors focus on procedural training. The trial-and-error instructors may unconsciously assume that by training learners on procedural practices, learners should naturally develop the specialist's mindset and associated moral behaviors pertinent to the specialist's role. The appropriately trained instructor, however, doesn't leave moral development to chance or allow learners to develop this on their own. As noted earlier, learners who develop their own explanations (in this case, explanations about the unique ethics of a specialty) often develop faulty thinking. Trained instructors combat learner errors by guiding and shaping explanations about underlying principles and beliefs by using well-defined training techniques. Techniques, such as cognitive apprenticeship, enable instructors to make the tacit explicit and thereby learnable.

Certainly, learned instructional capabilities through trial and error assumes a simple view of the instructional process. Such instructors may effectively develop learners toward becoming expert specialists, but the probability for learners to form faults or bugs in their thinking cannot be ignored. To decrease buggy thinking or the development of malrules related to ethical thinking and the specialist's mindset, accepting and acting from a more complex instructional model could help learners. Not only would this type of instructor become more effective and responsible in developing learners toward expertise, but they themselves develop a deeper and richer meaning about their specialty in terms of mindset and ethical thinking. Thus, such instructors become better care providers for patients as well as their learners.

Endnote

[1] Merriam et al. (2007) categorized the multiple learning theories into five orientations. The table below summarizes the purpose and instructor's role for each orientation.

Learning Orientation	Purpose	Instructor's Role
Behaviorist	To produce behavioral change in desired direction	Arrange environment to elicit desired response
Humanist	To become self-actualized, mature, autonomous	Facilitate development of whole person
Cogitivist	To develop capacity and skills to learn better	Structure content of learning activity
Social Cognitive	To learn new roles and behaviors	Model and guide new roles and behaviors
Constructivist	To construct knowledge	Facilitate and negotiate meaning-making with learner

Table i. Excerpt from Merriam et al.'s (2007) table entitled, "Table 11.1. Five Orientations to Learning" (295-96).

Second Edition Introduction References

In the introduction, I often refer to chapter authors from the book, *Knowing, Learning, and Instruction*. Rather than listing book repeatedly for each chapter, I list the chapters together:

Knowing, Learning, and Instruction: Essays in Honor of Robert Glaser (Psychology of Education and Instruction Series) (Ed L. B. Resnick). Hillside NJ: Lawrence Erlbaum Associates, Inc.,1989.

- Bereiter, C. and m. Scardamalia. "Intentional learning as a Goal of Instruction" 361-92.
- Brown, A. L., and A. S. Palincsarin. "Guided, Cooperative Learning and Individual Knowledge Acquisition" 393-451.
- Chi, M. T. H. and M. Bassok. "Learning from Examples via Self-Explanations" 251-82.
- Collins, A., J.S. Brown, and S. E. Newman. "Cognitive Apprenticeship: Teaching the Crafts of Reading, Writing, and Mathematics" 453-94.
- Gelman, R. and J. G. Greeno. "On the Nature of Competence: Principles for Understanding in a Domain" 125-186.
- Larkin, J. H. "What Kind of Knowledge Transfers?" 283-305.
- Nesher, P. "Microworlds in Mathematical Education: A Pedagogical Realism" 187-215.
- Resnick, L. B. "Introduction" 1-24.

Blanchard, K., and Garry Ridge. *Win at Work: A business Philosophy Called "Don't Mark My Paper, Help Me Get an A"*. Upper Saddle River, NJ: FT Press, 2009.

Bosk, C. L. *Forgive and Remember: Managing Medical Failure* (Second Edition). Chicago: The University of Chicago Press, 2003.

Groopman, Jerome. *How Doctors Think*. Boston: Houghton Mifflin Company, 2008.

Merriam, S. B., R. S. Caffarella, and L. M. Baumgartner. *Learning in Adulthood: A Comprehensive Guide*. San Francisco: Jossey-Bass, 2007.

Scarlett, H. *Neuroscience for Organizational Change: An Evidence-based Practical Guide to Managing Change*. Philadelphia: Kogan Page Limited, 2016.

Thalheimer, Will. *Performance-Focused Smile Sheets: A Radical Rethinking of a Dangerous Art Form*. Work-Learning Press, 2016.

Further reading about Bosk and Groopman

I accessed the following links on 15 November 2017:

Charles L. Bosk, Ph.D., Professor

Sociology at the University of Pennsylvania Faculty Page
https://sociology.sas.upenn.edu/c_bosk

ResearchGate Profile
https://www.researchgate.net/profile/Charles_Bosk

Jerome Groopman, Author, Physician, and Scientist

Author Homepage
http://jeromegroopman.com/

Author Wikipedia Entry
https://en.wikipedia.org/wiki/Jerome_Groopman

How Doctors Think Wikipedia entry
https://en.wikipedia.org/wiki/How_Doctors_Think

Introduction to the First Edition

In this qualitative study, I examined the clinical practice of family-practice specialists developing a specialty-interest area without becoming another type of specialist. My research question is:

> What type(s) of learning best explain how family-practice specialists engage in specialty-interest areas without becoming another type of specialist?

To address this question, I collected data from family-practice specialists in the Carle Clinic Association who were nominated or were self-nominated as having adapted to a specialty-interest area. To collect and interpret the data, I used the constant-comparative method of qualitative analysis.

Results from the analysis suggest that family-practice specialists are challenged by a three-way interlocking dilemma that influences how they learn and practice in specialty-interest areas such as sports medicine, obstetrics, occupational medicine, or even acupuncture and HIV counseling. The dilemmas are:

- Control vs. Autonomy
- Procedures vs. Invention
- Safe Practice vs. Risky Practice

Resolving each dilemma becomes imperative to handle the potential occurrences of untoward events successfully. Successful resolution entails consciously accepting both extremes of each dilemma while considering one as the syntonic and the other as the dystonic. This resolution leads to a broader awareness of the potential for untoward event development, risk management, rescue, and recovery of such occurrences.

While any modality of learning can be used to instruct non-risky procedures, only modalities that are grounded in social-cognitive learning can effectively and responsibly instruct clinical medical practices. The modality that best operationalizes social-cognitive learning is cognitive apprenticeship, which can be supplemented with microworld theory and the BOGERD technique.

Chapter 1

Socialization, Family Practice, and Specialty-Interest Areas

My research focus (depicted as "F" in Figure 1) is on clinical practice of specialty-interest areas by family-practice (FP) specialists who have entered a specialty-interest area without becoming another type of specialist. This type of clinical practice results from the socialization (depicted as "S1" in Figure 1) to a specialty-interest area without switching to another specialty after having been socialized to family practice.

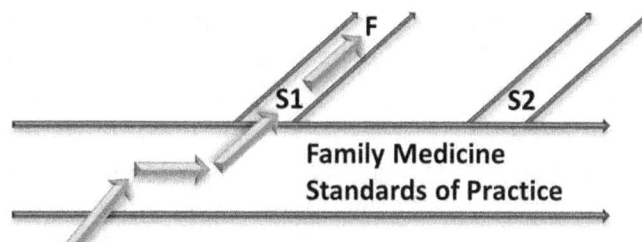

F = (Focus of the research project) Clinical practice of specialty-interest areas by FP specialists who have developed a specialty-interest area without becoming another type of specialist

S1 = Socialization to a specialty-interest area

S2 = Socialization to another specialization by switching specialties

Figure 1. Focus of the Research Project

Research Question

My research question of this study is:

> What type(s) of learning best explain how
> FP specialists engage in specialty-interest
> areas without becoming another type of
> specialist?

To address this question, I collected data from FP specialists in the Carle Clinic Association who adapted to a specialty-interest area without becoming another type of specialist. The clinic's education department nominated some of the FP specialists while other self-nominated. To answer the research question, relied upon a survey questionnaire, one-on-one interview, and document analysis.

Proficient Practice

The proficient practice (depicted as "P" in Figure 2) of a specialty-interest area is defined as handling specific types of situations using procedures, which are acceptable to family practice, a specialty-interest area, and/or another specialty. In other words, the procedures used comply with the gold standards (depicted as "GS1" in Figure 2) of family practice, of a specialty-interest area (depicted as "GS2" in Figure 2), and/or of another specialty (depicted as "GS3" in Figure 2).

Practice can be inconsistent with the gold standards of family practice (depicted as "B1" in Figure 2), of a specialty-interest area (depicted as "B2" in Figure 2), or of another specialty (depicted as "B3" in Figure 2).

Innovation (depicted as "I" in Figure 2) and research (depicted as "R" in Figure 2) may be engaged in by FP specialists and those FP specialists practicing in specialty-interest areas who are experienced and otherwise qualified to engage in such activities. Innovation and research may be used to discover new procedures or new applications for procedures. They may or may not subsequently be consensually validated by the profession, specialty, or specialty-interest area. If new procedures are confirmed in this way, they become new gold standards. Innovation is free-lance problem solving and, as such, is very different from using procedures that have been constructed and consensually validated by a profession, specialty, or specialty-interest area for use in dealing with a type of situation.

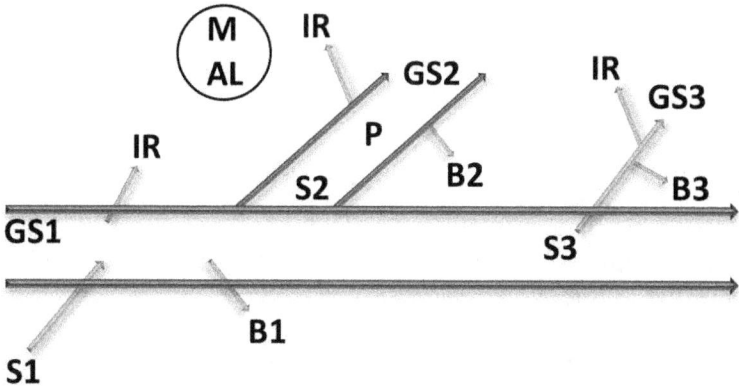

P   = Proficient practices by FP specialists who have gone into a spe-cialty-interest area without shifting to another specialty
S1 = Socialization of learners to family practice
S2 = Socialization of FP specialists to a specialty-interest area
S3 = Socialization to another specialty by switching specialties (e.g., FP specialist becoming an orthopaedic surgeon)
GS1 = Gold standards of FP
GS2 = Gold standards of a specialty-interest area
GS3 = Gold standards of another specialty (e.g., orthopaedic surgery)
B1 = Practice of family medicine inconsistent with the gold standards of family practice
B2 = Practice inconsistent with the gold standards of a specialty-inter-est area
B3 = Practice inconsistent with the gold standards of another specialty
AL = Adaptive leaders
M   = Models
I   = Innovation
R   = Research

Figure 2. Specialty-Interest Area as Emergent from FP (adapted from Handy, 1994 and Farmer, 1997)

Models (depicted as "M" in Figure 2) may or may not help FP specialists adapt to specialty-interest areas. Moreover, adaptive leaders (depicted as "AL" in Figure 2) may or may not help them switch from family practice to a specialty-interest area. Per Heifetz (1994), adaptive leadership entails the following:

- Finding opportunities and problems
- Adding or removing pressure
- Linking learners to resources
- Passing the ownership of the adaptive process back to the learners

Key Terms

Below are definitions of key terms related to how FP specialists socialize to specialty-interest areas. You can find these and additional terms in appendix I: Glossary.

Family Practice

Family practice is a medical specialty, which emphasizes "care of the individual, not as an isolated entity, but within the context of a family" (American Academy of Family Physicians, 1996). Family practice departments offer broad-based services, which are "not limited by a patient's age, sex, involved organ system or disease entity" (American Academy of Family Physicians, 1996). FP medicine emphasizes comprehensive care, preventive medicine, and patient education.

Family Practice (FP) Specialists

FP specialists are medical doctors, doctors of osteopathy, nurse practitioners, and certified physician assistants who have been socialized to and work in the family-practice field. FP specialists may also be those who now practices medicine in another specialty field in which the FP specialist has gone into a specialty-interest area. For example, doctors of osteopathy whose background is in family practice and who have gone into a specialty-interest area in orthopaedics would be of this type if they work in an orthopaedic department. This specialty-interest area may contribute to orthopaedics by giving a family practice and/or osteopathic perspective on types of orthopaedic medical cases.

Gold Standard

In the singular form, *gold standard* refers to the range of practice that a profession has found to be acceptable. Family practice, for example, has a gold standard that creates boundaries within which FP specialists can ethically practice (depicted as "GS1" in Figure 1). Working outside of this boundary (depicted as "B1" in Figure 1) generally is unacceptable and may threaten quality of patient care and may lead to litigation.

Gold Standards

In the plural form, *gold standards* refer to the procedures for dealing with types of medical cases that a profession, specialty, or specialty-interest area has constructed and gained wide acceptance (i.e., consensually validated). For example, there are gold standards for setting fractures and gold standards for conducting general physical examinations. These gold standards operate within the gold standard of the profession, specialty, or specialty-interest area.

Socialization

Socialization is an initiation process, part tacit and part explicit, into the elaborate and complicated environment of clinical practice. Socializing FP specialists to a specialty-interest area involves instructing specific knowledge and skills. Socialization involves acquiring the values and beliefs of the organization including:

- Ethics
- Power structures
- Roles
- Standing traditions
- The jargon (Anderson, 1994)

Specialty-interest areas

Specialty-interest areas involve finding a niche to make a valuable and sometimes unique contribution. Specialty-interest areas can play an essential complimentary role by bringing in what is

needed from another field and/or by offering services more economically. FP specialists can develop a specialty-interest area
within a department of family practice. They also can go into a specialty-interest area by finding a niche within another specialty area.

Proficiency

Proficiency is defined as the ability to handle a type of situation
using an acceptable procedure that has been constructed and consensually validated by one's profession, specialty, or specialty-interest area for handling such situations while avoiding unacceptable
practices (Lippert, and Farmer, 1984).

Background: Family Practice Specialization

Introduction

To understand better the phenomenon that I studied and to help
differentiate FP specialists from other types of medical specialists,
I describe the FP specialization in this next section.

Differentiating the FP Field from Other Specialties

FP medicine uniquely focuses on "the continuity of care and fam-
ily-oriented comprehensive care" *(Graduate Medical Education Directory*, 1997-1998, 69). While other primary-care specialists may
have a similar focus, only family practice offers an extensive, residency program that emphasizes this depth of holistic care (*The Directory of Family Practice Residency Programs*, 1996). Central to
proving successful, holistic care is the philosophy that FP specialists need to develop an intimate physician-patient relationship
(Roberts, 1995; Holleman, and Brody, 1995; Rakel, 1995). Rakel
(1995) states:

> The greater the degree of continuing in-
> volvement with a patient, the more capable
> the physician is in detecting early signs and
> symptoms of organic disease and differenti-
> ating it from a functional problem. Patients
> with problems arising from emotional and
> social conflicts can be managed most effec-
> tively by a physician who has intimate

knowledge of the individual and of his or her
family and community background. This
knowledge comes only from insight gained
by observing the patient's long-term patterns of behavior and responses to changing stressful situations. (7)

Specifically, FP specialists are trained to consider environmental, behavioral, and personal factors, which can critically effect the
patient's general health. Such training includes "taking into account
social, behavioral, economic, cultural, and biologic dimensions"
(*Graduate Medical Education Directory*, 1997-1998, 69). Specifically, FP specialists are trained to understand non-medical
knowledge in areas such as "family dynamics, interpersonal relations, counseling and psychotherapy." (Rakel, 1995, 3). The ethics
of family practice uniquely mandates that FP specialists:

...must help patients recognize, express,
and interpret their emotions...The physician
who ignores the emotions dehumanizes the
physician-patient relationship (Holleman,
and Brody, 1995, 159).

Specialty-Interest Areas and Sub-specializations

Critical for success in family practice is being socialized to a
comprehensive medical care that "spans the entire spectrum of
medicine." (Rakel, 1995, 9). This entails handling types of problems
that occur uniquely within any specific age group. Because family
practice emphasizes a holistic, broad approach to medicine, the
profession discourages sub-specializations. Per Rakel (1995), sub-
specialists limit their range of expertise to handle complex, ill-defined cases, which conflicts the functionality of primary practice.

FP specialists who engage in specialty-interest areas compliment general family practice. Because such FP specialists tend to
care for a wide-range of patients as well as focus on their specialty-
interest area, they continue practicing a comprehensive model of
care (*The Directory of Family Practice Residency Programs*, 1996).

Family Practice as a High-Risk Field

Part of the philosophy of family practice comes out of practicing within a high-risk field. As with other specialties, family practice is a high-risk field, which involves unique risks that can lead to untoward events. Roberts (1995) identifies these areas where FP specialists can experience untoward events:

- Failure to diagnose
- Failure to obtain informed consent
- Failure to obtain timely consultations
- Negligent obstetrical practices
- Negligent performance of a procedure
- Negligent treatment with drugs

While each category implies errors on the part of the FP specialists, Roberts (1995) acknowledges that even when FP specialists give optimal care, negative consequences still can occur.

To decrease untoward events, FP specialists are encouraged to engage in active risk management procedures as well as enhancing quality assurance (Roberts, 1995). *Risk management* is a set of procedures for finding, evaluating and correcting potential risks, which can cause harm to patients, professional staff, personnel and/or property (Anderson, 1994). *Quality assurance* involves dealing with common types of pitfalls that can occur within a procedure in which there are known ways for managing these pitfalls (Roberts, 1995). The cornerstone of medical risk management is reflective medicine. Roberts explains that FP specialists who uses reflective medicine "continuously recognizes medicine's ability to do harm, reflects on the patient's progress, and strives to keep the patient satisfied" (1678).

An example of a risk management procedure is crisis intervention in office practice (Feinstein and Carey, 1995). While many FP specialists may not consider themselves competent in crisis intervention, this model provides theory and a treatment plan, which can be implemented within time constraints of a general office practice in family medicine.

In addition to risk management, family practice emphasizes preventive medical procedures to diagnose illnesses and injuries in their early, undifferentiated state (Rakel, 1995). To be effective in this type of diagnosis, FP specialists needs to understand probabilities for types of problems occurring within the environment (the community that the FP specialists serve) as well as other environmental factors that might offer insight into potential illnesses and injuries, and that might hinder a patient's recovery (Rakel, 1995).

Chapter 2

Specialty-Interest Area Socialization Models

Inside-Out Doughnut Model

Handy's (1994) inside-out doughnut model graphically explain Specialty-interest areas. The conceptual model depicts a shape resembling a doughnut with the hole is on the outside and the dough or solid-part is in the middle. In this model (depicted as Figure 3), the core of the doughnut holds the practice in keeping with the gold standards of family practice.

While many specialists learn to become an expert in the core or the heart of the doughnut (Handy, 1994), some choose to expand their core to include a specialty-interest area. Per Handy, the core is not the whole doughnut. What lies beyond the core are the degrees of freedom for adapting or shifting to a specialty-interest area.

Vygotsky (1992) describes this outer region of Handy's inside-out doughnut as the zone of proximal development. The zone of proximal development is the extent to which FP specialists can potentially adapt to a specialty-interest area without becoming another type of specialist. Handy (1994) characterizes this space as "our opportunity to make a difference, to go beyond the bounds of duty, to live up to our full potential" (70). The zone of proximal development (depicted as "ZPD" in Figure 3) is the extent to which FP specialists can potentially expand their abilities within family practice and their specialty-interest areas.

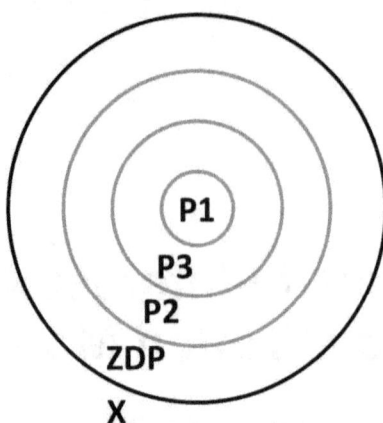

P1   = Practice in keeping with the gold standards of FP
P2   = Practice in keeping with the gold standards of a specialty-interest
          area
P3   = Practice in keeping with the gold standards of another specialty
ZPD   = Zone of proximal development
X   = Practicing outside the zone of proximal development

Figure 3. Specialty-Interest Areas as Depicted Using Handy's Inside-Out
          Doughnut Model

Practicing beyond the outer circle (depicted as "X" in Figure 3) of the inside-out doughnut without shifting to another type of specialty is illegal, irresponsible, and/or fraught with intolerable risks (from the perspectives of patients, the medical profession, and society).

Cardiology Specialty-Interest Area Example using Handy's Inside-Out Doughnut Model

Sam, a FP specialist, chose to develop a specialty-interest area in cardiology without becoming a cardiologist. Rather than formally entering a cardiology residency, Sam retains his FP specialty while emphasizing cardiology procedures within his practice. To do so, Sam must socialize (depicted as "S2" in Figure 2) to the new specialty-interest area's gold standards (depicted as "B" in Figure 4) while continuing to practice within the gold standards of family practice (depicted as "A" in Figure 4). In addition, Sam has Yolanda, a cardiologist, help him learn specific procedures typically done by cardiologists in keeping with their gold standards of cardiology (depicted as "C" in Figure 4). For some time, Sam works under the ongoing auspices by Yolanda. With her support, Sam learns to handle some types of situations proficiently using procedures that are in keeping with the gold standard of family practice, his specialty-interest area, and cardiology. That intersection is depicted as "D" in Figure 4.

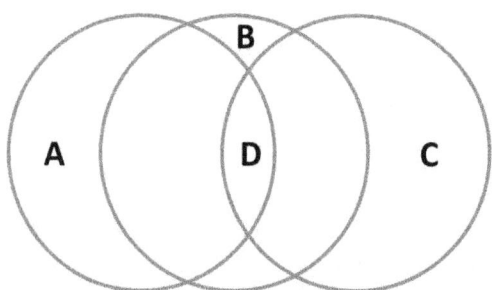

A = Gold standards of FP
B = Gold standards of new specialty-interest area in cardiology within FP
C = Gold standards of cardiology
D = Commonality between the gold standards of FP and of cardiology

Figure 4. Example Relationship of Cardiology Specialty-Interest Area in FP

Socializing to a specialty-interest area involves more than learning to do additional procedures in keeping with the gold standards of the specialty-interest area or another specialty. This involves developing a distinct worldview (Kekes, 1980) or paradigm (Kuhn, 1970) that gives a unique outlook. As depicted in Figure 4, the gold standards of the specialty-interest area of cardiology include primarily the gold standards of family practice, and secondarily, the gold standards of cardiology.

Specialty-interest areas entail assimilation or accommodation. If the FP specialist handles a situation from a FP perspective with modification, assimilation is occurring. If he handles a case from another perspective, then accommodation occurs.

Alternative Scenarios for Specialty-Interest Areas

FP specialists can go into a specialty-interest area and continue practice in the FP department or can practice in another department. They can also switch to another specialty. Some FP specialists can stay within the field of family practice while treating patients who see them for their proficiency in their specialty-interest area. Such FP specialists may work in a FP department and have other FP specialists consult with them about cases that fall under their specialty-interest area. Likewise, FP specialists may receive internal referrals related to their specialty-interest area.

Other FP specialists that develop a specialty-interest area may work within another specialty department. Such professionals would not behave as a specialist from that field per se but would instead work with patients using the specialty-interest area's procedures as well as their FP procedures. For example, a doctor of osteopathy who may have started working in a FP department might shift to working in an orthopaedic department. Unlike that department's orthopaedic surgeons, the doctor of osteopathy doesn't handle complex surgical cases that require expertise in orthopaedics. Rather, the doctor of osteopathy may evaluate patients and use procedures in osteopathy to help patients in ways that an orthopaedic surgeon can't. In this way, they contribute to orthopaedic medicine. The FP specialist may also perform orthopaedic procedures under supervision, such as carrying out certain injections, handling sprains, and other similar types of medical cases.

Some FP specialists may enter a second residency program (depicted as "S3" in Figure 2) and become socialized to the gold standards of that field (depicted as "GS3" in Figure 2). For example, Susan, a FP specialist, develops an interest in psychiatry. She has a strong interest for handling different types of depression, but she recognizes that diagnosing depression can be complicated and, at times, inaccurate (Mintzberg, 1996). Because Susan is unsatisfied with keeping the specialty-interest area, she decides to enter a psychiatry residency program.

As stated earlier, specialty-interest areas are done either through assimilation or are done through accommodation. This process may or may not involve the socialization of new FP specialists who develop a specialty-interest area. Such socialization results in their practice within and supported by a cadre of FP specialists that go into the same specialty-interest areas rather than developing individualistic, free-lance specialty-interest areas from the perspective of family practice.

With these alternatives, FP specialists shift from the FP gold standards to a new specialty-interest area's gold standard. This is done by working within the area of the outer doughnut (that I described earlier). FP specialists expand their core to assimilate or to accommodate to the specialty-interest area's gold standards, which determines the degree of the shift.

As Handy (1994) explains, working in the outer area of the doughnut involves specialists encountering complex problems. Handy warns that facing complex problems is high risk, but high risks are necessary to develop the specialists' abilities and necessary to satisfy the specialists' responsibility and duty to treating patients. By engaging in a specialty-interest area within family practice, FP specialists can better meet the needs of patients and improve the quality of patient care in general.

Explaining Specialty-Interest Areas Using Handy's Sigmoid Curve Model

An adaptation of Handy's sigmoid curve explains how the gold-standards of specialty-interest areas occur (depicted as Figure 5). Handy characterizes the life-span of an individual, organization or society in terms of the sigmoid curve. Like a sigmoid curve, an individual's career can wax and wane. The length of a sigmoid curve varies from individual to individual.

In Figure 5, the beginning of the first sigmoid curve can be interpreted in terms of the gold standards of family practice in which a FP specialist begins to consider developing a specialty-interest area. As FP specialists socialize to the FP gold standards, they reach a point in which they become proficient in diagnostic and treatment of FP procedures (depicted as "A" in Figure 5). Thus, they work within the gold standards of family practice.

In area "B" of Figure 5, FP specialists enter the *dark woods*. Handy describes the dark woods as a time of initial exploration and floundering in which there is confusion in adapting to the second curve.

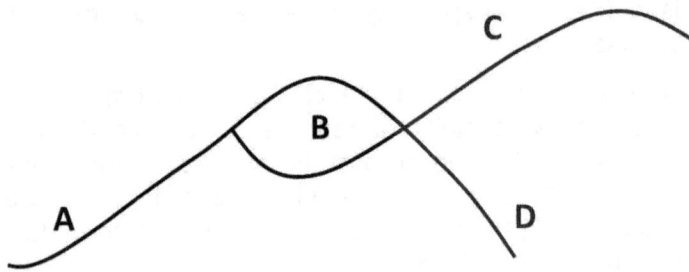

A = FP specialist practicing proficiently within the gold standards of
   family practice
B = Dark Woods
C = FP specialists practicing proficiently within the gold standards of fam-
   ily practice, this new specialty-interest area, and/or another specialty
D = Practicing inconsistent with relevant gold standards

Figure 5. Explanation of the Process of Specialty-Interest Areas Using
      Handy's Sigmold Curve

Because of internal or external pressures, FP specialists face
the dilemma of adapting or not adapting to the second curve. Internal pressures such as boredom of routine, personal interest, or desire to develop new opportunities or talents, which are not fully experienced in family practice (such as surgical skills), and ethical issues may drive them into the dark woods. External pressures (such
as organizational changes, shifts in managed-care policies, and encouragement from supervisors, colleagues, experts, and consult-
ants) may likewise drive them into the dark woods.

Because the second curve (gold standards of the specialty-interest areas) is different from the first curve at point "A" (proficiently
practicing the gold standards of family practice), proponents of a
strict form of family practice may pressure FP specialists into the
dark woods by discouraging them from developing a specialty-interest area. FP specialists in the dark woods need to cope with negative as well as positive pressure when contemplating whether to
shift to the second curve (depicted as "C" in Figure 5).

After overcoming these types of pressures, FP specialists begin
the second curve and develop a specialty-interest area within family

practice. At "C" in Figure 5, FP specialists socialize to the new specialty-interest area. They adapt to a different set of gold standards. They also may become part of a cadre of FP specialists within a specialty-interest area who function proficiently in keeping with the gold standards of that specialty-interest area. As FP specialists within that area, they may deal with types of situations using procedures that have been constructed and consensually validated by their primary specialty (i.e., family practice), by their specialty-interest area, or by another specialty. Practices inconsistent with relevant gold standards are sub-standard. This is depicted as "D" in Figure 5.

In summary, the second curve differentiates FP specialists who engage in the practice of a specialty-interest areas. For example, a FP specialist who develops a specialty-interest area in orthopaedics didn't train as extensively or intensively as orthopaedic residents, and cannot practice the orthopaedic worldview or paradigm.

To engage in a specialty-interest area of orthopaedics, FP specialists can no longer view orthopaedics in the same way as other FP specialists. Handy (1994) explains that the second curve (representative of specialty-interest areas) is different from the first curve (representative of the FP field) for development to occur. To become proficient in specialty-interest areas, FP specialists must practice and adapt to new sets of gold standards.

Summary

In this chapter, I described two models and give examples to describe how socialization to specialty-interest areas work:

- Handy's Sigmoid Curve
- Handy's Inverted Doughnut

I also discussed Vygotsky's Zone of Proximal Development and Heifetz's Adaptive Leadership.

Chapter 3

Types of Learning and Training Techniques Used in Professions

Introduction

Medicine is a high-risk field (Bandura, 1986). Medical specialists function under real-life time constraints in which actions taken, not taken quickly enough, or omitted may lead to harmful consequences. Patients may experience complications, emotional or physical distress, or even loss of life if they don't administer the proper procedures. Because high-risk fields must compensate for potentially causing harm when learning the gold standards, Bandura (1986) argues that professionals in high-risk fields must learn differently from learning in low-risk fields. Bandura argues that learning in high-risk fields is best handled with social-cognitive learning. This type of learning minimizes the potential for causing harm by eliminating trial-and-error learning. Despite Bandura's argument, other form(s) of learning may, in fact, be used as a primary method in each circumstance. These other types of learning may even realistically compliment or supplement social-cognitive learning for proficiently helping specialists learn in high-risk fields.

Social-cognitive learning

Introduction

Social-cognitive learning presupposes a triadic reciprocal model (as depicted in Figure 6) consisting of behavior, personal factors (cognition), and environmental events (social) perform as interacting determinants of each other for explaining human function (Bandura, 1986).

Reciprocity does not imply symmetry in strength of influence. At times, environmental events may have a dominant influence over behavior and personal factors. For example, a FP specialist may develop a specialty-interest area due to strong environmental events (such as an adaptive leader putting pressure on the FP specialist to shift to the second curve) despite behavioral and personal factors. Per Bandura, when situational constraints are weak, personal factors become predominant. Hence, if there are no adaptive leaders pressuring for FP specialists to develop a specialty-interest area, and if there are no external pressures (such as a FP specialist who finds a need for specialty-interest areas in family practice or is under administrative pressures to do so), then the choice of develop a specialty-interest area rests upon personal factors (such as interest in pursuing more surgical proficiencies or pursuing additional sports medicine experiences).

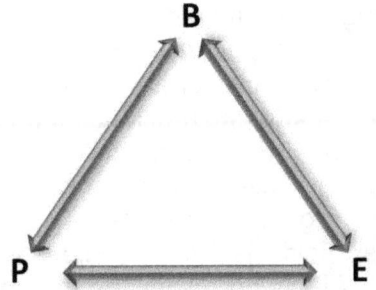

B = Behavior
P = Cognition and Personal Factors
E = Environmental Conditions

Figure 6. Social-Cognitive Learning Theory's Model for Triadic Reciprocal Causation

Five Capabilities of Personhood

Based upon the model of triadic reciprocity, Bandura identifies five, basic capabilities for describing the nature of personhood.

Capacity 1: Symbolizing capability

By using symbols, individuals can process transient experiences into internal models (Bandura, 1986). These models can help an individual in preparing for future actions. Symbols give meaning, form, and continuance to one's situational experiences. They help individuals to alter and adapt to their environment.

As stated earlier, a paradigm or worldview (for example, interpreting medicine from the viewpoint of family practice, orthopaedics, or pediatrics) defines a specialist's scope of practice. Certain symbolic structures of a paradigm determine how specialists define their scope of practice, determine the procedures of that paradigm, and determine how they perceive a given medical case. An emergency room physician may examine a patient much differently than a primary care physician due to time constraints or the function of different protocol.

Another benefit of symbolizing is the capacity to test potential solutions symbolically rather than enacting options that may entail costly missteps. Thus, Bandura (1986) writes:

> An advanced cognitive capability coupled
> with the remarkable flexibility of symboliza-
> tion enables people to create ideas that
> transcend their sensory experiences. (18)

Symbolism is the basis for scaffolding in cognitive apprenticeship. With scaffolding, the learners practice a procedure within controlled conditions so that no harm occurs. For example, a FP resident may practice procedures on a cadaver before doing so on patients.

Bandura (1986) cautions that individuals may fail to behave objectively rational. In trying to understand a phenomenon symbolically, errors can occur when trying to actualize the procedure. Bandura (1986) states:

> Even if people know how to reason logically,
> they make faulty judgments when they base
> their inferences on inadequate information
> or fail to consider the full consequences of
> different choices. Moreover, they often
> miss-sample and misread events in ways
> that give rise to erroneous conceptions
> about themselves and the world around
> them. (19)

This relates to the applicative fallacy (Farmer, 1997). The applicative fallacy involves applying a procedure, for example, after having only read about it. What may not have been conveyed in the text are:

- Underlying principles
- Potential pitfalls
- Heuristics or tricks-of-the-trade

Social-cognitive learning attempts to avoid this fallacy through cognitive apprenticeship (as I discuss later).

Capacity 2: Forethought capacity

Rather than at once reacting to an environment or being driven by past behaviors, most individuals try to regulate behavior by using forethought (Bandura, 1986). By expecting potential consequences, individuals set goals, avoid ineffective choices, and anticipate consequences of actions. FP specialist can use forethought to evaluate how a medical case is proceeding. FP specialists then can modify what treatments to use based on the patient's progress.

Capacity 3: Vicarious capability

Per Bandura (1986), all learning phenomena based upon direct experience can occur vicariously through observation. An individual can observe another person's actions and further see the results of those actions. Bandura states:

> The capacity to learn by observation enables people to acquire rules for generating and regulating behavioral patterns without having to form them gradually by tedious trial-and-error (19).

Bandura warns that trial-and-error learning can lead to costly mistakes. When the potential for costly and hazardous mistakes is high, learners must rely more on observational learning from competent models.

Capacity 4: Self-regulatory capability

An important feature of social-cognitive learning is self-regulatory capability. Per Bandura (1986), much of human behavior is motivated and regulated by internal standards and self-evaluative responses:

> Thus, by arranging facilitative environmental conditions, recruiting cognitive guides, and creating incentives for their own efforts, people make causal contribution to their own motivation and actions. (20)

Capacity 5: Self-reflective capability

This capability enables learners to interpret their experiences and evaluate their own thought processes. By doing so, learners shift from different perspectives when analyzing an experience (Bandura, 1986).

Social-Cognitive Learning Techniques

Social-cognitive learning can be used in high-risk professions in the form of cognitive apprenticeship (Brandt, Farmer, and Buckmaster, 1993). Instructors can supplement cognitive apprenticeship with the concepts of microworlds, constructive and destructive bugs (Burton, Brown, and Fisher, 1984), and the BOGERD technique (Bulstrode, and Hunt, 1997). I discuss these below.

Cognitive-Apprenticeship Technique

Cognitive apprenticeship (Collins, Brown, and Newman, 1989; Farmer, Buckmaster, and LeGrand, 1992; Brandt, Farmer, and Buckmaster, 1993) operationalizes social-cognitive learning through the usage of five phases, which I outline in appendix A. By using these sequential phases, cognitive apprenticeship gives a systematic method for socializing learners to procedures from the gold standards of family practice, a specialty-interest area, or another type of specialty.

Cognitive apprenticeship involves focusing on types of situations rather than specific individualistic problems. Training involves modeling the proper procedure as defined by the relevant profession applied to a specific type of situation.

Listed below are the five phases of cognitive apprenticeship. All phases are necessary for training.

Phase one: observation with articulation

In the first phase, the primary activity is having models, as described by Lave and Wenger (1991), who are proficient in handling types of situations in proper ways as defined by the gold standards. The trainers or proficient specialists do the modeling. Sometimes trainers are merely resource linkers and process facilitators if they are not themselves proficient in the procedure being instructed. The learners' role is to observe the model performing the proper procedure for handling a type of situation. The procedure is performed in a real-life, clinical setting which situates the experience. While performing the procedure, the model articulates the underlying principles and heuristics or tricks-of-the-trade that make the procedure work, pitfalls to avoid, which can get learners in trouble, and risk management.

The model identifies the pitfalls that are likely to give a procedure and situations difficulties. The model explains how to spot and avoid them, and the model describes the constructed way to manage them when they do occur. Thus, the model articulates risk management procedures which have been consensually validated by the field as proper ways to manage pitfalls for the type of situation.

Phase two: scaffolding and coaching

The purpose of phase two is to allow learners to model a procedure under controlled conditions. These conditions are known as scaffolding (Rosenshine, and Meister, 1992). Learners must approximate doing the real thing while articulating aloud the principles, heuristics or tricks-of-the-trade, and risk management to the trainer. As needed, the trainer clarifies these principles, heuristics, and risk management and offers support. Trainers use scaffold conditions to minimize harm. Thus, performing a procedure on a cadaver, for example, might be necessary to prevent potential harmful effects on live patients and to allow for appropriate coaching to occur.

Phase three: fading

In phase three, the principle concept is to have the model fade by decreasing the amount of coaching and scaffolding. Learners continue to approximate the real procedures under supervised conditions. Instructors can do this either in groups or individually. Models continue to offer support and coaching when needed and continue to ensure that learners follow the procedures as defined by the gold standards rather than to allow them the opportunity to invent on their own.

Phase four: Internalization

Learners, in this phase, internalize the modeled procedure. Models allow learners to personalize the procedure (Bandura's personal factor element of the triadic reciprocal causation model) to make what they do as their own but only within the constraint of the gold standards as defined by the profession.

Internalization involves learning the procedure in ways that are situationally appropriate. Making the procedure work well for themselves and be situationally proper must be done within the limits which are acceptable to the field. This is analogous to what Thompson (1993) refers to as bounded flexibility. Learners don't end up engaging in self-directed learning or an autonomous practice in phase four of cognitive apprenticeship. Rather, they engage in proficient practice in which they perform the procedure that has been constructed and consensually validated by the profession or the FP specialists in the specialty-interest area in ways that work for them and are situationally appropriate.

Phase five: Generalizability

This phase involves having the trainer provide an advanced organizer (West, Farmer, and Wolff, 1991). To do so, the trainer reviews the main principles underlying the modeled procedure and explains how those principles are used in similar procedures, which the trainee has yet to learn. Trainers also not differences among the procedures. Advance organizers can be used to identify what is yet to be learned, which employ heuristics or tricks-of-the-trade as well as risk management techniques associated with the modeled procedure.

By engaging in this phase, trainers bridge or link what has been learned to new situations, thus giving a structure for learning how to handle similar types of problems. West et al. (1991) state that the key to this phase is the similarities between the procedures learned and specific ones yet to be learned. Without substantial similarity, the advanced organizer cannot work.

Microworlds and Constructive/nonconstructive Bugs

Burton, et al. (1987) operationalize social-cognitive learning through the concept of microworlds and constructive/nonconstructive bugs. I discuss both next.

Microworlds

Per Burton et al. (1987), the learning process can be conceptualized as increasingly complex microworlds. Trainers present specific types of situations or *microworlds*. The trainer models how to handle the microworld by applying proper procedures, as defined by the gold standards of family practice, the specialty-interest area, or the specialty. After the learners handle the microworld proficiently, the trainer presents a similar but more complex microworld and models how to handle it using relevant gold standard procedures. Learners, again, practice under guidance on proficiently use the procedures for handling the microworld. Upon being proficient with this microworld, the trainer shifts to an even more complex one. By doing so, the trainer is bootstrapping (Resnick, 1989) the learners within their zone of proximal development (Vygotsky, 1978) so that they can handle more complex microworlds, and thus expand their central core to include a specialty-interest area of those types of microworlds.

Constructive/nonconstructive bugs

Per Burton et al. (1987), all microworlds, including well-defined ones, have constructive and nonconstructive bugs. These bugs are pitfalls that can get the practitioner in trouble if not handled appropriately as defined by the profession. *Constructive bugs* are pitfalls that learners can handle. *Destructive bugs*, which Burton et al. (1987) identify as *Nonconstructive bugs*, are pitfalls that learners are not able to handle on their own nor can they be instructed to handle them responsibly at this stage of their professional develop-ment. Thus, destructive bugs fall outside of the learners' zone of proximal development.

Training microworlds include constructive bugs so that learners can become proficient in dealing with them. Trainers should avoid presenting microworlds which have destructive bugs. To teach such a microworld would be unethical and cause harmful consequences to patients.

BOGERD Technique

The BOGERD technique, designed by Bulstrode and Hunt (see discussion of this technique in Lippert, Farmer, Murnaghan, and Sarwark, 1997) is a supplementary process for cognitive appren-ticeship. BOGERD contributes to cognitive apprenticeship and is a conceptual way of contracting meaningful supervised medical edu-cation. This technique focuses on a clinical procedure and the proper time constraints.

The BOGERD technique has been adapted for use in cognitive apprenticeship (Lippert e al, 1997) to ensure that trainers meet the clinical learning needs and to ensure that responsible risk manage-ment takes place to protect patients, as much as possible, from un-toward events.

BOGERD is an acronym for which each letter stands for a phase of the sequential process. Phases one and two need to occur before the other phases. Phases three, five and six occur before cognitive apprenticeship starts. The fourth phase occurs throughout the train-ing process. Before using BOGERD, the trainer selects a focal pro-cedure that is part of the gold standards of the profession. Upon identifying this procedure, the trainer proceeds with the first phase of BOGERD.

Background

Clinical educators need to ascertain the nature and extent of prior medical education and experiences relative to the procedure to be learned. The trainer does this by asking the learners questions about their background and experiences with this procedure and other similar ones. Trainers might also determine this background based on examining any personnel files, if ethically available for review.

Opportunity

In this phase, the trainer finds any foreseeable opportunities for supervised educational experiences in relation to cognitive apprenticeship. Thus, the trainer needs to decide, based on the background of the learners, whether modeling is needed (learners may have already had the procedure modeled sufficiently but haven't performed the procedure). If phase one of cognitive apprenticeship is not needed, the trainer needs to figure out which subsequent phases of cognitive apprenticeship would offer opportunities for the learners. Such experiences may include:

- Having the learners apply the procedure to cadavers
- Using the procedures to help patients but under guidance of the trainer
- Require the trainer to discuss the generalizability of what was previously learned as it applies to other procedures (i.e., phase five of cognitive apprenticeship).

Goal

The goal of professional training is for trainers to socialize learners to the gold standards of their specialty-interest area. While there is overlap between the gold standards of family practice and of a given specialty-interest area (such as the gold standards of family practice and gold standards of obstetrics), the specialty-interest areas' gold standards "tend to differ and are subject to change over time in response to forces that are internal and/or external to the profession and due to contributions of clinical, epidemiological, and basic science research" (Lippert et al., 1997, 45).

Evaluation

Lippert et al. (1997) explain that the evaluation phase is extremely important. Trainers need to decide how and when the learners are to be evaluated, especially because evaluation varies from phase to phase in cognitive apprenticeship. At the end of phase one, the trainer needs to decide whether the learners are prepared to continue to phase two. Thus, the trainer needs to check whether they learned enough from observation and listening before starting to phase two.

In phase two, the trainer needs to offer relevant feedback, as needed, in the forms of suggestions and feedback to ensure that the procedure is performed correctly. The trainer also needs to summatively evaluate the learners. That is, based on their current performance, the trainer needs to let learners know if they can continue with the procedure. If not, the trainer needs to help the learners by modeling and articulating again. At the end of phase two and three, the trainer needs to alert the learners whether their clinical performance merits the decreasing amount of coaching and scaffolding.

In conducting evaluations, Lippert et al. (1997) recommend using Pendelton Rules. These rules occur in six sequential steps:

1. The trainee is asked what he/she thought went well.
2. Then the trainer is asked the same question.
3. Next, the evaluator says what went well.
4. The trainee is asked what could have been done better.
5. The trainer is asked the same question.
6. The evaluator comments on what he/she thinks could have been done better. (46)

Rescue

For responsible scaffolding to occur and minimize risks, the trainer must develop a rescue plan of action. *Rescue* can be defined as:

> ...a plan of action, understood and agreed upon by the trainer and trainee, about who is to do what if things go wrong when the trainee is doing the clinical procedure throughout Phases #2-4 in cognitive apprenticeship. (Lippert et al., 1997, 46)

Deal

This is a formal agreement between the trainer and the learners, which states explicitly who performs what roles and when they are to be performed within the five phases of cognitive apprenticeship.

Reception and Autonomous Learning

In addition to social-cognitive learning, I found that reception and autonomous learning to be relevant in my research. I described these next.

Reception Learning

Another type of learning is reception learning. This type of learning involves "reading, hearing or observing what is to learned much in the form in which it is to be received" (West et al., 1991, 253). Reception learning assumes that there is a trainer of some type giving the necessary information. Reception learning is one-directional learning in which the learner receives the information in this way in which it is intended to be used. An assumption in reception learning is that the learner will be able to understand the instruction given and can apply what has been received.

Autonomous Learning

Ausubel, Novak and Hanesian (1978) describe autonomous learning as a self-discovery process. In this approach, learners seek to develop procedures independently rather than receive instructions from another person. Autonomous learning does not involve reading of materials but does involve inventing procedures through trial-and-error.

Autonomous learning should not be confused with the fourth phase of cognitive apprenticeship. Internalization is not synonymous with autonomous learning. Internalization involves finding ways to make a procedure work for learners but within the limited boundaries of the field's gold standards. Invention is not part of internalization.

Autonomous learning is different from self-directed learning. Per Candy (1991), self-directed learning is an umbrella term that may include the following:

- A method for organizing one's choice of training
- Autonomous learning
- Intellectual pursuits
- Internalization
- Reading self-selected materials
- Self-actualization activities
- Solitary activities

Because of the wide-range of activities associated with this term, self-directed learning cannot be a single modality of learning.

Bandura (1986) cautions against trial-and-error approaches due to potential harm one can cause patients. Likewise, Ausubel et al. (1978), warn that autonomous learning works only for certain specified situations and purposes:

> Learning by discovery is simply not a feasible primary method of transmitting large bodies of subject-matter content (for learners who are capable of learning concepts and principles through expository teaching) to warrant the vastly increased time-cost it entails. (520)

Additional Training Techniques

Guided Inquiry Technique

Per Gagne (1985), guided inquiry is characterized as a form of learning which is learner-driven and in which the learners discover how to solve problems. This approach leverages reception learning and autonomous learning (West, et al. (1991). There are six phases to this approach:

Phase 1.   The first phase is for the trainer or both the trainer and learners to identify the presenting problem for which they will address.

Phase 2.   Once this is identified, the learners with or without the trainer decide the intended goals for the exercise.

Phase 3. The learners try to array relevant concepts that might help the learners in achieving the intended goal of the learning experience.

Phase 4. The learners then systematically relate the identified problem with each of the relevant concepts in an experimental manner. This is done under the guidance of the trainer who acts as a coach for the learners. As the learners apply a concept, the coach might inform the learners whether they are getting closer or farther away from solving the problem. For example, the coach might tell the learners that they are getting warmer or colder. This process continues until the learners solve the identified problem and has the "Ah ha!" experience.

Phase 5. The product and process are evaluated either by the trainer alone or with the learners.

Phase 6. The learners and trainer discuss the experience.

While cognitive apprenticeship socializes learners to the gold standards by focusing on types of situations and how practitioners from the field proficiently handle those types of situations, guided inquiry focuses on specific problems and allows for invention through trial-and-error. While guided inquiry may promote effective innovations, innovations are discouraged if the innovations conflict with existing procedures that have been consensually approved by the profession for handling such types of situations. Moreover, Landa (1983) states that guided inquiry tends to be too time-consuming for learning established procedures.

Guided Shaming Technique

A dysfunctional form of guided inquiry is guided shaming (Resnick, 1989). This form of guided inquiry is negative and punitive and consists of setting the learner for failure. In guided shaming, the trainer encourages the learners to begin a task for which they are not developmentally ready to accomplish in a satisfactory manner. Upon failing partially or completely, the trainer salvages and completes the task. Resnick (1989) explains that guided shaming can result in the following:

- Decreased motivation
- A downward shift in the learners' learning curve
- If the learners arrive at a partially satisfactory completion of the procedure, integration of the unsound conclusion

Resnick (1989) argues that trainers have a more difficult time in getting learners to unlearn misinformation and inappropriate usage of procedures than to teach learners the acceptable ways (as defined by the profession) for handling types of situations.

Socratic Learning Technique

Socratic learning (Segen, 1992) is an alternative teaching philosophy that instructs learners to invent ways of handling types of problems rather than having trainers socialize new learners to gold standards. Socratic learning involves having trainers ask questions designed to elicit contradictory inferences to eliminate inappropriate principles and procedures and to bring about the proper ways of handling certain types of situations. In doing so, instructors allow learners to invent their own methods for handling types of situations which, in turn, encourages learners to use them to handle other types of situation when they are on their own.

Socratic learning encourages learners to develop individualistic innovations rather than practice consensually validated procedures by the profession.

Segen explains that the Socratic method is most effective in oral examinations and least effective for aiding in standardized examinations.

Sequencing Types of Learning

Sequencing types of learning can strengthen the quality (West et al, 1991). To illustrate this, suppose that Jan, FP specialist in sports medicine, wants to learn how to manage complex fractures that occur on a playing field. If Jan has a solid understanding of fractures, she might start with reception learning in which she reads journals, listens to some lectures, and observe how other FP specialists manage such fractures. This is pure reception learning.

If Jan assumes that she can figure out on her own how to apply what was learned (inventing how to do so on her own), then she is using autonomous learning.

Instead of autonomous learning, suppose that after Jan reads, listens, and observes how others handle complex fractures, Jan receives coaching from Scott, an established FP specialist in sports medicine, and does this under scaffold conditions and before Jan handles actual cases, then she is experiencing social-cognitive learning. Specifically, Jan experiences cognitive apprenticeship phases two and three. Thus, Jan uses reception learning followed by social-cognitive learning phases two and three.

If an established Scott occasionally helps as needed, then Jan experiences the fourth phase of cognitive apprenticeship.

If Scott helps Jan understand how to make the procedure work best for her by asking her questions, then Scott is helping Jan internalize the procedure (phase four of cognitive apprenticeship).

Sequencing learning can help learners improve how they apply the principles, protocols, and cognitive thinking when practicing the procedures. Complementing types of learning, such as cognitive apprenticeship with reception learning, also can enhance the quality of learners' experience.

Summary

In this chapter, I introduced the phenomenon that I studied and presented the relevant educational theories for understanding an overall framework of types of learning. The types of learning are:

- Autonomous learning
- Guided inquiry
- Guided shaming
- Reception learning
- Social learning theory
- Socratic method

I explained how types of learning can be sequence is given as well as an explanation on how to differentiate the different types.

In the next chapter, I explain the focus of this study, the research question, variables to answer the research question, relationships between those variables, and the methodology I used for this study.

In this section, we explain the focus of this study. The research question enables us to answer the research question, resolution, which leads to the experimental design.

Chapter 4

Methodology: Qualitative Approach, Site Selection, Data Collection, and Analysis

The focus of this research is clinical practice of specialty-interest areas by FP specialists who have entered a specialty-interest area without becoming another type of specialist. The research question of this study is:

> What type(s) of learning best explain how FP specialists engage in specialty-interest areas without becoming another type of specialist?

In this chapter, I describe my method for data collection and data analysis. I discuss concerns and techniques for controlling the this process. Specifically, I describe:

1. The timeline for the research project
2. Research strategy and ethical concerns
3. Choice of methodology
4. Choice of the site location
5. Explanation of how I collected data
6. An explanation of how I analyzed data

Timeline of Activities

Figure 7 describes my sequence of activities. I used this functional flowchart as a guideline for accomplishing specific tasks. The arrows show the relationships between the activities. For example, the results from the literature review influenced how I collected data, analyzed and interpreted the data, and wrote about the study. At the same time, information from the interviews produced a need for more searches in the literature.

Activity	Time Period (October 1997 through April 1998)				
	October November	December January	February	March	April
Written Products					Dissertation
Committee Meetings	Preliminary Oral				Final Oral
Survey		X			
Individual Interviews		X	X	X	
Document Analysis	X	X	X	X	
Analysis of Data	X	X	X	X	
Interpretation of Data	X	X	X	X	
Literature Review	X	X	X	X	

Figure 7. Timeline of Activities

Research Strategies and Ethical Considerations

I incorporated research strategies that I identified for this qualitative approaches. Researchers use these strategies as guidelines to figure out appropriate procedures. Zelditch (1962) names two primary criteria for keeping realistic and proper procedures. Zelditch calls the first criterion *Information Accuracy*. This criterion states that the research project must be constructed to maximize the opportunities for the researcher to thoroughly, precisely, and accurately understand the context of the phenomenon. Preventing this criterion from being taken to an unrealistic extreme is the second criterion, efficiency. Efficiency involves developing a research plan that enable researchers to collect data adequately but with the minimal amount of cost. Cost can be construed as the amount of time needed to gather data, as the extent of access to the setting and research respondents within that setting, and as the degree of time spent with research respondents.

Limiting the extent of applying these two criteria are ethical considerations. Per Marshall and Rossman (1989), ethical considerations are critical for judging the extent of designing research strategies. Researchers decide how much a research project can disrupt a research respondent's activities. This must be a priority for the researcher. Likewise, researchers determine the extent in which research respondents are placing themselves at risk by taking part in the study. Corollary to this is the researcher's determination of whether the research strategies could cause a violation of human rights in some manner.

In considering the criteria for research strategies and ethical considerations for this research project, I collected data using a variety of techniques including:

- Literature review
- Document analysis
- A survey questionnaire
- One-on-one interviews

I used this variety of techniques for gathering data to meet the information accuracy criterion. I assumed that each technique gives a more accurate and thorough understanding of the phenomenon when used in conjunction versus only using one technique alone. To meet the criterion of efficiency, I collected data in a short period. To decrease intrusion, I used a survey questionnaire to answer preliminary questions about the phenomenon and to find potential candidates for individual interviews. I present the survey in appendix D.

For ethical considerations, I designed techniques to protect research respondents by ensuring anonymity. If, for example, the data from the surveys indicate that research respondents would be at risk if they were involved in a focus group, then I wouldn't use focus groups and would conduct individual interviews instead. Because the American Academy of Family Practice do not certify the development of specialty-interest areas, there is a possibility that research respondents may be at risk if I named them within the study. Secondly, if the nature of the data is controversial, research respondents may withhold data when among their peers within a focus group. If I expect this, then focus groups would be contraindicated as per the information accuracy criterion as well as by ethical considerations. If, however, this were not the case, I would use focus groups because focus groups are an effective and accurate manner for gathering data from groups of research respondents. As a group, respondents are more likely to accurately describe the phenomenon than any given individual (Senge, Kleiner, Roberts, Ross, and Smith, 1994). Thus, in this case, criterion of information accuracy would be met without violating ethical considerations. Because of the lack of willingness of the respondents, and because of the considerable distance between the different respondents, I decided that a focus group was contraindicated. Instead of using a focus group method, I chose to use one-on-one interviews as the primary collection technique.

In developing collection techniques for any research project, research strategies, and ethical considerations should become a critical factor in designing collection techniques. When identifying specific questions for survey questionnaires and individual interviews, information accuracy, efficiency, and ethical considerations will help keep appropriateness in research design of such instruments.

Qualitative Research as Methodology

Schumacher and McMillan (1993) state that, while quantitative research attempts to figure out relationships and explain causes of changes in measured social facts, qualitative research focuses on understanding social phenomenon from the participants' perspectives. Qualitative method enables researcher to develop an understanding of the language and assumptions held by research respondents. This method also helps researchers understand how respondents assign meaning to situations encountered in their work setting (Sommers, 1997). Biklen and Bogdan (1986) call this "thinking naturalistically," a process by which researchers try to understand how different stakeholders perceive the meaning of behaviors around them. They further argue that the ways in which research respondents interpret and assign meaning to experiences, behaviors and events will determine how they will act within their given setting. Qualitative method tries to explore the research respondents' point of view to explain behavior. Per Krathwohl (1993), such studies result in context-dependent and sometimes multiple explanations that usually are written as a case study involving one or more sites.

Because this research project is not designed to explain causal relationships, I didn't use a quantitative method. Rather, a qualitative method is a proper approach for understanding this phenomenon because of the emphasis on understanding how FP specialists perceive their development and learning experiences. Secondly, because one of my objectives is to derive meaning in how the field of family practice changes within the modern healthcare context, I decided that a qualitative method would be effective in reaching this objective.

Exploratory approach

Marshall and Rossman (1989) state that exploratory studies can be used "to investigate little-understood phenomena, to identify/discover important variables [and] to generate hypotheses for further research" (78). Per Sommers (1997), researchers should use an exploratory approach when investigating little-understood phenomena, for finding or discovering meaningful variables, or for generating new hypotheses for future research. Exploratory research can subsequently benefit by finding important variables (Marshall, and Rossman, 1989). Exploratory research is thus needed where researchers have not found or recognized relevant variables as well as where researchers don't know the tacit elements of organizational behaviors. Because specialty-interest areas have not been extensively studied considering the current changing healthcare environment, I chose to use an exploratory approach to find relevant variables of the educational process, and for building a rich, thorough description of this complex process.

Constant-Comparative Method of Qualitative Analysis

Introduction

The constant-comparative method is a means for not only processing data but for deriving grounded theory (Lincoln and Guba (1985). Glaser and Stauss (1973) describe the purpose of this method is to generate theories in a systematic way by using explicit coding and analytical procedures. Data collected are not extensive enough to test or to discover theory, but only to suggest and generate potential theory. Glaser and Strauss (1973) state:

> The constant comparative method is concerned with generating and plausibly suggesting (but not provisionally testing) many categories, properties, and hypotheses about general problems...Some of these properties may be causes, as in analytic induction, but unlike analytic induction others are conditions, consequences, dimensions, types, processes, etc. In both approaches, these properties should result in an integrated theory. Further, no attempt is made by the constant comparative method to ascertain either the universality or the proof of suggested causes or other properties. Since no proof is involved, the constant comparative method in contrast to analytic induction requires only saturation of data – not consideration of *all* available data, nor are the data restricted to one kind of clearly defined case. (104)

The constant-comparative method can produce discussional or prepositional theory (Glaser and Strauss, 1973). These types of theories are useful in that they can easily be translated into formal hypotheses for testing purposes.

Constant-Comparative Method in Contrast with Quantitative Experimental Studies and Non-Experimental Naturalistic Studies

In contrast with this approach are quantitative experimental studies and non-experimental naturalistic studies. Quantitative experimental studies use statistics to show what is significant or important beyond the level of chance. Non-experimental naturalistic studies involve the researcher collecting data (data by means of a questionnaire or an interview process) followed by having the researcher quantify that data. Researchers then decide what is important, usually through descriptive statistics, where it is assumed that more is necessarily better, or through inferential statistics, where research-ers show the extent which things vary beyond the level of chance.

These two approaches are not right for this study due to the na-ture of the research question; however, the constant-comparative method is. This approach, recommended by Lincoln and Guba (1985), is a non-numerical approach to analyze and interpret natu-ralistically obtained data. Per Glaser and Strauss (1973), this ap-proach is appropriate for use when the main research question is not focused on *how many* or *to what extent*, but *what kind(s) or type(s)*, as is the case with the main research question for this study:

> What type(s) of learning best explain how
> FP specialists engage in specialty-interest
> areas without becoming another type of
> specialist?

Site Selection

To understand the phenomenon that I studied, I describe the Carle Clinic Association in this section. The site I selected for this research project is the FP department in the Carle Clinic Associa-tion.

The Carle Clinic Association, which is one of the largest private physician groups in Illinois, runs the second largest outpatient facil-ities within the state. There are over 50 medical and surgical spe-cialists and sub-specialists employed by the clinic. While the clinic is primarily found within the main hospital in Urbana, Illinois, the clinic runs 12 branch clinics throughout the Central Illinois. Sites include Bloomington, Mahomet, Champaign, Mattoon, Danville, Monticello, Farmer City, Rantoul, Georgetown, Southeast Urbana, Gibson City, and Tuscola. All of them have FP departments, and most branch clinics operate within a rural community. Most of the respondents work in the branch clinics.

The main hospital in Urbana also supports two residency pro-grams, namely FP Residency and Internal Medicine Residency. Be-cause most of the branch clinics are found within a rural setting, residents in family practice can enter the Rural Training Track through which additional training in orthopaedic care, emergency medicine, and trauma are offered. Those residents who want a more obstetrical experience for their future practices can receive more training in this area.

In addition, the Carle system supports training for third, and fourth year medical students attending the University of Illinois at Urbana-Champaign. All physicians within the clinic are considered members of this teaching faculty for the residency programs and for the medical students. Both residents and medical students rotate through various departments found at the main hospitals and at the branch clinics.

Data collection

Introduction

Using complementary data collection techniques is highly recommended for improving the understanding of the phenomenon (Green (1997). Jonassen, Hannum, and Tessmer (1989) state that there are several complementary techniques that can be used for collecting data. For this research project, I used the following techniques: document analysis, survey questionnaires, and one-on-one interviews.

Key Informants

The key informants were those in the Carle-Clinic administration who are aware of FP specialists who engage in specialty-interest areas. I selected key informants based on the recommendations of the director of the FP attendings.

The key informants named the specialty-interest areas for which they were aware of in family practice. They then ranked them as well as recommend FP specialists from the Carle system who are practicing within a specialty-interest area. I discuss the results from the key informants in chapter 3.

Survey Questionnaires

The second step of this research project was to conduct a survey of all FP specialists within the Carle system. I didn't make the survey anonymous so that I could conduct follow-up, one-on-one interviews. I kept all information confidential and coded. Rather than to collect statistical information, the purpose of the survey was to find FP specialists who have engaged in specialty-interest areas. I asked respondents who indicated on the questionnaire that they have a specialty-interest area to specify this on the questionnaire:

1. The nature of their specialty-interest areas
2. The percentage of their practice time devoted to the practice of a specialty-interest area
3. If they would be willing to take part in a one-on-one interview or a focus group.

I didn't include demographics as part of the survey due to the nature of the main research question and due to the requirements of conducting a constant-comparative method of qualitative analysis.

Sampling

From the Carle System, I interviewed two key informants and 15 FP specialists. The key informants, described in chapter 3, referred the 15 FP specialists as well as the categories of specialty-interest areas. The other respondents consisted of 12 physicians, two nurse practitioners, and one certified physician assistant. I list in Table 1 the different specialty-interest areas of the FP specialists.

In this table is the frequency of FP specialists per specialty-interest area. The total frequency of specialty-interest areas is greater than those interviewed due to one FP specialist having two specialty-interest areas and another having three.

Specialty-Interest Area	Number of Respondents
Sports Medicine	Four
Occupational Medicine	Three
Adolescent Medicine	One
Obstetrics	One
Women's Health	One
Adult Medicine	One
Geriatric Medicine	Two
Public Health	One
Acupuncture	One
Emergency Medicine	One
HIV Counseling	One
Psychology or Counseling	One

Table 1. Specialty-Interest Areas and Number of Respondents Per Area

One-on-one Interviews

Jonassen, Hannum, and Tessmer (1989) state that the purpose for the interview technique is "to seek the advice of expert performers or respondent matter experts on various dimensions or components of a task." To do so, I adopted a form of elite and specialized interviewing from Dexter (1970). While the survey only gave basic information about FP specialists and their specialty-interest areas, using Dexter's (1970) elite and specialized interviewing technique provided details including a richer description of FP specialists educational process, problems or concerns with that process, and more details about their current practice. Dexter describes this type of interview as follow:

> [An elite interview] is an interview with any
> respondent – and the stress should be on
> the word "any" – who in terms of the current

purposes of the interviewer is given special, non-standardized treatment. By special, non-standardized treatment I mean:

1. stressing the respondent's definition of the situation
2. encouraging the respondent to structure the account of the situation
3. letting the respondent introduce to a considerable extent (an extent which will of course vary from project and inter-viewer to interviewer) his notions of what he regards as relevant, instead of relying upon the investigator's notions of relevance

Put another way, in standardized interview-ing – and in much seemingly non-standard-ized interviewing, too (for instance, in Mer-ton's "focused interview" in its pure form) – the investigator defines the question and the problem; he is only looking for answers within the bounds set by his presupposi-tions. In elite interviewing, as here defined, however, the investigator is willing, and of-ten eager to let the respondent teach him what the problem, the question, the situation is – to the limits, of course of the inter-viewer's ability to perceive relationships to his basic problems, whatever these may be.

In standardized interview, the typical survey, a deviation is ordinarily handled statistically; but in an elite interview, an exception, a de-viation, an unusual interpretation may sug-gest a revision, a reinterpretation, an exten-sion, and a new approach. In an elite inter-view it cannot at all be assumed – as it is in typical survey – that the persons or catego-ries of persons are important. (5-6)

Data Analysis

Introduction

Data collection and data analysis occur simultaneously and is an emergent process (Petry, 1991). Merriam (1988) describes the collection/analysis process in the following way:

> Analysis begins with the first interview, the first observation, the first document read. Emerging insights, hunches, and tentative hypotheses direct the next phase of data collection, which in turn leads to refinement or reformulation of one's questions, and so on. It is an interactive process in which the investigator is concerned with producing believable and trustworthy findings. (119-120)

Although data collection and data analysis occur simultaneously, data analysis doesn't end when researchers collect all data. Rather, analysis becomes more intensive after researchers gather the data (Merriam, 1988).

In this section, I discuss analysis during data collection and analysis after data collection. I analyzed the data using the constant-comparative method. This analysis process is like content analysis, as described by Merton (1968). Per Merton (1968), content analysis consists of the following:

1. Symbol counts, which consist of identifying and counting substantial symbols from the one-on-one interviews and focus group sessions, if any

2. One-dimensional classification of symbols, which involves classifying the key symbols in accordance to how they are used

3. Item analysis, which consist of classifying divisions of the interview sessions in which significant and insignificant items are distinguished based on the study's theoretical foundation

4. Thematic analysis, which involves classifying implicit and explicit themes from the interview sessions

5. Structural analysis, which pertains to examining key-interview themes and distinguishing complementary from interfering relationships

From the data analysis, I placed specific attention on finding any dilemmas and/or paradoxes, which might exist in the respondents' practices and within the process of becoming proficient in the clinical practice of specialty-interest areas. I discuss in chapter 4 implications for handling such dilemmas and/or paradoxes.

Analyzing Data During Collection

Introduction

Analysis is an ongoing process throughout the research project. Without continuous analysis, researchers could easily run into the pitfall of collecting unfocused, repetitious, and overwhelming data. Data that is analyzed as it is collected can be illuminating (Merriam, 1988). As with a formative evaluation (West, et al., 1991), once a collection situation has occurred, researchers figure out from the analysis how to improve future collection situations.

Nine Suggestions for Analysis During Data Collection

Merriam (1988) discusses nine suggestions devised by Bodgan and Bilken (1982) for analyzing data during the collection period. I used these suggestions as guidelines for both data collection and analysis for this research project. Listed below are the nine suggestions, and I explain how I integrated this into my research.

Suggestion one

Researchers need to discipline themselves into making decisions that narrows the study. Researchers who pursue too many potential interests could derive data that is inappropriate and too diffuse. By limiting the range of the topic or setting, researchers are more capable of developing deeper analysis.

With this research project, instead of examining all primary care specialists (i.e., internal medicine and pediatrics), I focused on FP specialists. Each FP specialist was unique in how he or she learned their specialty-interest area, how they interact with other specialists (e.g., patient needs of children are much different than those of older adults), and how they interact within their group. Limiting the research respondents to FP specialists helped limit the range of variation within these variables.

Suggestion two

Researchers need to force themselves to make decisions concerning the scope of the study. By deciding whether to perform a full description of the study or one aspect of it, researchers develop a clearer focus for analysis.

During data collection, analysis from the data helped me narrow the research scope. As I gathered data, research respondents helped me improve my focus. Thus, limiting the study's focus helped make the data collection process more efficient and effective.

Suggestion three

Researchers formulate analytic questions before data collection. While collecting data, questions should be reexamined to determine how appropriate they are given new insight from the phenomenon. Questions should be reformulated to direct future data collection better.

Based upon the literature, I present a set of research questions in chapter 3. I summarize these questions in appendix E. As I gathered data, I considered each question to figure out the relevancy in light on data collected as well as determine which questions I need to be reformulate. I discuss this revision in chapter 3.

Suggestion four

Researchers use collected data to plan future data collection opportunities. For example, an interview may offer insight into understanding the phenomenon, which enables for more accurate interviews regarding specific issues or respondents.

As I collected data, I found lessons learned from each data collection session to improve on the accuracy of future data collection sessions. Improvements included asking more specific and relevant interview questions.

Suggestion five

During data collection, researchers should write as many observer comments as possible. The purpose is to stimulate critical thinking about observations during data collection.

I used this by keeping detailed field notes. At the end of an interview, I quickly wrote in a journal a summary of what occurred as well as initial thoughts about the session. Likewise, after listening to the audiotape, I added to the journal any new insights or impressions.

Suggestion six

Researchers need to write memos about what they learn from the data collection. Unlike the earlier suggestion, this focuses analysis on a meta-level in which researchers consider how the data relates to theoretical and methodological issues.

While collecting data for this project, I compared how collected data relates to what the literature discusses. For example, I considered how Handy's (1996) sigmoid curve related to how FP specialists engaged in specialty-interest areas. I illustrate this example in chapter 4.

Suggestion seven

Researchers should present themes or ideas to respondents for feedback. While this may not work well for all research respondents, some may be able to advance analysis and fill in gap descriptions.

I benefited by presenting ideas and themes to FP specialists during interviews. When I asked respondents if a particular theory described accurately their learning experiences, or when I asked respondents to reframe the theory by describing it in their own words, their responses helped me understand how FP specialists perceived their specialty-interest areas.

Suggestion eight

Researchers continue to explore the literature on that field. Not only does new studies become available which can add insight into data collection, but researchers can expand their understanding of what to look for due to being more familiar with the phenomenon.

During the data collection, I continuously reviewed the literature.

I also asked respondents if they are aware of any writings, which offered some insight into how FP specialists develop specialty-interest areas.

Suggestion nine

Researchers may get stuck by "nearsightedness." To encourage thinking about the phenomenon in different ways, Bodgan and Bilken (1982) suggest trying to apply metaphors, analogies or other concepts to descriptions about the phenomenon.

Types of Learning and Their Functions

I developed Table 2 for analyzing data from the one-on-one interviews. This table is a specification table for classifying types of learning.

Summary of Analysis During Data Collection

By using Bodgan and Bilkens' (1982) suggestions for analyzing data during collection, I improved the quality of the data collection. Analysis and collection should be more efficient and effective. By continuously analyzing the data while collecting, I had a better understanding of the data when I completed collection and began my intensified analysis.

Data Analysis After Collection of Data

Introduction

After collecting data, the process of analyzing the data becomes intensified (Merriam, 1988). Researchers bring together all documentation, memos, fieldnotes, transcripts, and questionnaires to begin organizing the material so that they could readily access data (Yin, 1984). In this section, I explain how I organized the data and what came from this process.

Three Categories of Analysis

Per Petry (1991), data analysis is an interactive process consisting of three simultaneous activities: data reduction, data display, and data conclusions. I describe these three activities below. With each activity, I explain how I integrated the concept to my research.

Function	Cognitive Apprenticeship	Guided Inquiry	Autonomous Learning	Reception Learning
Modeling	Yes	No	No	Sometimes
Articulation (talking out loud and explaining principles, tricks, and risk management)	Yes	Yes	No	Sometimes
Coaching	Yes	No	No	No
Scaffolding	Yes	No	No	No
Fading	Yes	No	No	No
Internalization	Yes	No	No	No
Generalization	Yes	No	No	No
Feedback	Yes	Yes	No	No
Invention	No	Yes	Yes	No
Observing	Yes	No	Sometimes	Sometimes
Reading	Yes	Yes	Yes	Sometimes
Listening	Yes	Yes	Sometimes	Sometimes
Socratic Dialogue	No	Yes	No	No
Talking through a Procedure	Yes	No	No	Yes
Hands-on Training	Yes	Yes	Sometimes	No
Trial-and-Error	No	Yes	Yes	No

Table 2. Types of Learning and Their Functions

Data reduction and content analysis

Data reduction is the process of selecting, focusing, simplifying, abstracting and trans-forming raw data that appear in written field notes." (Petry, 1991, pg. 56)

Data reduction begins with the design of the research project including:

- The development of the conceptual framework
- Research questions
- Collection methodologies
- The site chosen

This process continues by analytically coding and categorizing data as researchers collect them and after as well.

Although data reduction occurs throughout the process, I increased this activity after I collected data. Once I grouped data together, I analyzed the content using a constant-comparative method of qualitative analysis to examine data to find patterns that generate a theory or theories of how a social group functions. Marshall and Rossman (1989) describe this technique as an art that enables researchers to arrange categories to best help readers to understand the data. This involves coding data to help researchers find patterns that may not be clear to those within the social group or by outside observers. Marshall and Rossman state:

> ...it is a technique for making inferences by objectively and systematically identifying specified characteristics of messages. It is a way of asking a fixed set of questions about data in such a way as to produce countable results. (98)

Marshall and Rossman describe the following steps for conducting content analysis:

1. Researchers should set specific objectives for the analysis. This can include the objectives of "producing descriptive information, cross-validating research findings, or testing hypotheses" (99). With the constant comparative methodology, the objective is the research questions.
2. Researchers next need to locate relevant data and determine an empirical

link between the data that are identified and inferences to be made from the data. Specifically, researchers will need to develop a rationale to explain why the data relates to the objectives or research questions. Presenting relevant theories or models from the literature review to support linking data sets to specific research questions typically does this.

3. The next step is to devise a plan for identifying representative samples of possible data. This involves developing "a coding or classification system for analyzing the content" (99). Optimally, the researcher will want to use coding systems from previous research to save time and to utilize systems that have already been tested. Marshall and Rossman caution that defining content categories based on previous research is a critical step for making a contribution to the field under investigation.

4. The last step is for the researchers to report the frequency of the classification. For example, this research project may find that all research respondents use some type of autonomous learning and reception learning (two of the types of learning) for developing their specialty-interest areas. However, because constant comparative method was used to analyze the data, no frequencies were reported. This last step represents a traditional content analysis. This step is described here only to distinguish traditional form of content analysis from the constant comparative method (98).

In addition to constant-comparative method, Farmer, Gilbert, Murray, Snellen, Bragg, Deschler, and Paprock (1991) name three critical steps that compliment this method. First, the researchers should use an inductive approach for analyzing data so that they can classify data into categories or patterns. Second, researchers need to review each category for potential subcategories, possible relationships to other categories, and for recognizing any relationship to the whole. Lastly, researchers should continue the topical analyses among the categories.

Data display

Data display is the process of organizing information about the data in the form of tables, matrices, and other visual presentation. The purpose is to visually present the categories studied. This process is a technique for displaying triangulation by comparing data from different sources.

West et al. (1991) discuss cognitive strategies for displaying and arranging data. Cognitive strategies help researchers in managing complex information. Specific strategies include chunking, frames, and concept maps. I used these techniques to design the appendixes.

Chunking strategies involve organizing concepts as described by content analysis. Chunking information into groups help researchers deal with the complexity of the data. Chunking can be spatial, narrative, procedural, expositional, taxonomies, typologies, or multipurpose. Multipurpose sorting includes causes and effects, similarities and differences, forms and functions, and advantages and disadvantages.

Frames are matrices designed for representing knowledge.

Concept maps are visual graphics, which display concepts and relationships between those concepts.

Drawing conclusions

This process "begins when the data show evidence of the phenomena, regularities, patterns, explanations, or some relationship among variables" (Merriam, 1988, pg. 56). The development of theories is tentative while collecting data, and researchers may change findings as researchers discover new data.

Because purpose of the constant-comparative method is to generate theoretical ideas in the form of suggestions, the theories that I present in chapter 4 are not extensive enough to offer proof as to the generalizability. Such theories are only relevant to those whom I interviewed.

Line of Inquiry

I implemented this study in conjunction with a larger inquiry into how professionals learn and instruct high-risk work. I developed this line of inquiry in conjunction with other researchers and as an extension of earlier research found in the literature. My contribution offers examples of how FP specialists received training, learned, or experienced a combination of the two for developing their specialty-interest areas in the context of high-risk work. From my analysis, I discovered a complex dilemma and the importance of resolving that dilemma.

In addition, other researchers who were part of this line of inquiry focused on different training environments:

- Simulators: Green, 1998; Sommers, 1997
- Telemedicine consulting: Higgins (1998)
- Rehabilitation: Williams (1998)
- Child case work supervisions: Wehrmann (in progress)
- Orthopaedic surgery: Farmer (1997)

Summary

In this chapter, I described the method for collecting and analyzing data. This included the use of a survey questionnaire, one-on-one interviewing, and document analysis. I explained how I analyzed and interpreted the data.

Chapter 5

Stories about Learning Specialty-Interest Areas and the Findings

The research question of this study is:

> What type(s) of learning best explain how FP specialists engage in specialty-interest areas without becoming another type of specialist?

To address this question, I designed several subsequent questions to capture the complexity of specialty-interest areas (see appendix E). In this chapter, I describe:

1. The respondents
2. Findings from key informants
3. Findings from the survey questionnaire
4. Findings from one-on-one interviews for those who have developed specialty-interest areas
5. Three distinct patterns of relationship
6. Summary of the types of learning
7. Evidence of issues for learning specialty-interest areas

In this chapter, I state each question followed by a description and examples of responses from the respondents. As noted later in this chapter, I reframed certain questions to elicit responses from different perspectives.

Respondents

As described in chapter 2, I collected data from FP specialists who engage in a clinical, medical practice within the Carle Clinic Association and who developed specialty-interest areas. I collected empirical data through one-on-one interviews. Respondents included:

- 12 physicians
- Two nurse practitioners
- One certified physician assistant

All Respondents have formal training in family medicine and have developed specialty-interest areas. Two additional respondents were key informants.

Findings from Key Informants

Two physicians acted as key informants by nominating other FP specialists who were known for adapting to a specialty-interest area without becoming another type of specialist. Both key informants named the main types of specialty-interest areas and those practitioners in the Carle Clinic system who have gone into them.

The key informants further discussed what they would not consider to be a specialty-interest area. For example, under typical conditions, physicians would not develop a specialty-interest area in a type of disease or illness. Because of the number of accessible specialists and the limited number of cases for an injury or illness, physicians would have a difficult time maintaining and dedicating the time to become an expert in one type of illness or injury. One key informant, however, noted that exceptions might occur under certain conditions. For example, in a small mining town, a physician may need to develop a specialty-interest area in lung disease, especially if other types of specialists are not easily accessible in that area to handle such cases.

For the key informants, a specialty-interest area needs to compliment or supplement the FP field. One key informant said the following:

> Family practice is a broad specialty, and I'm
> not anxious to see it grow into a sub-spe-
> cialty field. Sub-specializing limits oneself
> and may interfere with the retention of the
> broad scope of procedures that such spe-
> cialists need to utilize in clinical practice.
> Look at what has happened in internal med-
> icine. That field has sub-specialized to the
> degree that physicians may not be qualified
> for general practice.

Thus, if FP specialists develop specialty-interest areas ethically, they should complement or supplement the broad scope of services of family practice. One key informant said:

> Physicians tend to forget what they don't
> practice. So, family-practice physicians
> need to maintain their practice in a variety of
> areas to keep current rather than focusing
> on one area of medicine.

Findings from Survey Questionnaire

I conducted a survey of all FP specialists within the Carle system to allow for self-nomination. In appendix D, I provide a copy of the survey questionnaire. Three FP specialists responded to this survey. I interviewed two of them.

Based on the low percentage of responses to the questionnaire, I decided that self-nomination using a survey questionnaire was an ineffective technique of finding potential respondents. For this study, I found potential respondents through key informants. Particularly important was the key informants' willingness to have their names used with those whom they identified. I used the following wording that worked particularly well in getting potential respondents to agree to be interviewed:

> I am a doctoral candidate at the University
> of Illinois currently conducting my thesis
> study under the supervision of Professor
> James Farmer and Dr. Terry Hatch. In dis-
> cussing my thesis with Dr. [key informant's
> name], Dr. [key informant] commented that

you have a specialty interest in [name of the specialty-interest area] and recommended that I interview you as part of my study.

Findings from One-on-one Interviews of Those Who Have Developed Specialty-Interest Areas

Introduction

Respondents practice medicine in a variety of specialty-interest areas. Their specialty-interest areas are the following:

- Acupuncture
- Adolescent medicine
- Adult medicine
- Emergency medicine
- Geriatric medicine
- HIV counseling
- Obstetrics
- Occupational medicine
- Psychology or counseling
- Public health
- Sports medicine
- Women's health

Before the interviews, I prepared nine questions to understand the phenomenon of going into specialty-interest areas within family practice and to explicate aspects of the research question within the phenomenon. I list these questions in appendix E. I used questions that appear in appendix E throughout the interviewing if the questions resulted in collected data needed to answer the research questions. Otherwise, I reframed the questions as needed. In appendix F, I list a copy of this revised interview schedule with reframed questions replacing original ones.

In the questions that follow, I give examples of typical responses for each category. I note any exceptions.

Question One: What Type of Work Do You Do?

To understand the scope of duties involved in practicing within specialty-interest areas, I asked respondents to describe their current work that they do within their clinical practice. Respondents described their departmental affiliation and explained they entered specialty-interest areas.

Departmental Affiliation

Respondents expressed that physicians and physician assistants who have gone into specialty-interest areas and remain in a FP department still considered themselves to be general practitioners or to be FP specialists rather than sub-specialists. While they worked many cases related to their specialty-interest areas, they kept a broad family practice. One physician, who has a specialty-interest area in geriatrics, still has patients who are children, adolescents, young adults, and middle-aged adults. He said:

> It was never my intention to sub-specialize in geriatric medicine. I think of myself as a general practitioner. I took the certificate of added qualification to increase my knowledge and ability to add to the care of elderly people. So I did this partly as an academic exercise; but, because I did receive the certificate, I decided to use this to my benefit. (Depicted as "5" in Table 5)

Because of the certificate in geriatrics, he works more in the elderly community than most FP physicians do. There are seven FP specialists who are affiliated exclusively with a FP department.

FP specialists may work part-time in a FP department and part-time in other specialty departments. Physicians who do this still align themselves with family practice. One stated, "Although I see a number of cases in occupational medicine, I still have my family practice."

Nurse practitioners who work full-time in other specialty departments don't consider themselves as FP specialists. Rather, they are practitioners who have learned to apply their FP knowledge and skills to a specialty department. One respondent said:

I consider myself to be an adult provider
who just happens to have a family nurse
practitioner's background. Because I haven't worked with children or in obstetrics
for so long, I really don't feel qualified to do
general practice.

Although this respondent works in adult medicine, she still discusses problems that FP specialists encounter:

In my first position, I spent time working with
family planning, underprivileged black com-
munities, teenage pregnancy, and public
health. Now I work more with counseling
HIV patients.

Why FP Specialists Enter Specialty-Interest Areas

There are four general reasons for FP specialists entering specialty-interest areas. First, personal factors can influence entering
an area. I found five FP specialists as this type. One respondent
said, "I've always had an interest in sports medicine. Over time, I
gradually grew interested in this area." Another FP specialist entered his specialty-interest area because of the challenges that the
area offers. He said:

I got into geriatrics because I found it to be
a stimulating, exciting practice. Because
others saw this in me, they encouraged me
to pursue this work. What fascinates me is
that one of the principles of geriatrics, which
is not part of family practice, has to do with
the non-presentation of disease. The patient
can be a little bit off mentally or a little bit
weaker, which can be an indication that
there is pneumonia. And they are not even
coughing! They don't even have a fever.
This is the challenge that I enjoy, and I enjoy getting into a whole new area of
knowledge and learning! (Depicted as "14"
in Table 5)

A second reason involves environmental and external factors that can influence this decision. Four FP specialists entered specialty-interest areas due to environmental factors. For example, a respondent said, "I had to move to the Champaign area. This position was available, and it suited my needs." Another stated, "There was someone who encouraged me to work with the elderly."

A third is behavioral factors, which describes two FP specialists. A respondent explained:

> I prefer to deal with instant reward. Shocking someone in arrest and bringing them back alive is an example of what I mean. Dealing with chronic diabetics who won't stay on their diets is not gratifying. These long-term cases were too frustrating for me in family practice. I needed something more rewarding. (Depicted as "8" in Table 5)

The fourth reason is a combination of the earlier three. I classified four FP specialists as this type. For example, one respondent said, "They needed a director for this specialty area. Because I was wanted to work with this population, I agreed."

Question Two: How Experienced Are You in Your Specialty-Interest Area?

There are three broad categories of responses to this question: well established, established, and getting started. I discuss each below.

Well-Established in Specialty-Interest Areas

Respondents considered those who received certificates of added qualification in a specialty-interest area without taking part in an internship or fellowship and had at least five years' experience in a specialty-interest area as being well established. I classified eight FP specialists as being well-established. Some may have helped pioneer their specialty-interest areas. One physician, for example, who practices in occupational medicine, said that he could not find mentors or help in applying what he had learned from family practice to an industrial environment. That respondent said:

I had to rely on the notes of the previous physician who worked here to help me figure out what I was doing. It was baptism by fire.

Established in Specialty-Interest Areas

Respondents considered FP specialists with two to five years of experience as having an established practice within their specialty-interest area. While the basis of practice comes from the FP residency programs, much of the situated learning occurs in clinical practice. I classified four of the FP specialists as established. One established physician said, "While I can handle most cases, I'm still gradually expanding the type of cases that I do."

Getting Started in Specialty-Interest Areas

Respondents considered those with less than two years' experience as just getting started in their specialty-interest area. I classified three FP specialists as getting started. One physician interviewed has practiced medicine for less than one year after residency. Most of what he does in his specialty-interest area came from his rotation in sports medicine. He said:

In my residency program, there was a particular sports medicine doctor that I worked with. I basically use what I learned from my interactions with him in my current practice.

Question Three: Is the Clinical Practice of Your Specialty-Interest Area Considered to be Risky?

To find the types of risks involved in developing and practicing a specialty-interest area, I asked respondents if they considered their specialty-interest area to be risky. When I said the question in this way to the first two FP specialists, both respondents denied that they engaged in risky work or were unsure. They claimed initially that, because they could apply procedures, which identify and bypass some pitfalls, they avoid risky problems. One physician explained, "I try not to think about possible risks." Only after further probing did he acknowledge that medicine could be risky but downplayed that risk.

A nurse practitioner reported that the protocol and supervision by physicians protects her from risk. She said:

> One of the ways that we safeguard us is that we are trained to operate under protocol. We can do things that are defined by our protocol and as defined by our physicians. Also, particular departments will have quality assurance guidelines set to protect us from errors. For example, every time that a patient is seen for the first time, the chart had to be reviewed by a physician. Every time I changed a medication, a physician would review that too. (Depicted as "1" in Table 3)

Because the nurse practitioner performs procedures and is closely supervised by physicians, she believes that practice in her specialty-interest area is safe.

To avoid the initial denial of risks, I reframed the question as follows:

> If errors occur within a procedure and/or if unforeseen events complicate a procedure, can untoward events occur?

Untoward events are circumstances that result in loss of life or limb, litigation, or loss of professional reputation. Untoward events can result from health providers making technical errors, judgmental errors, normative errors, or quasi-normative errors (Bosk, 1979). Untoward events, however, can occur because of pitfalls or other undesirable events, which were not caused by FP specialists. Such events may or may not be associated with health-provider errors. Bosk (1979) describes medical decisions as being a probabilistic enterprise in which there is often low-control over the circumstances. Bosk (1979) states:

> Only rarely is it the case in which the physician can say "this patient has x and we must do y." Even when it is certain that a patient has x, this does not dictate what should be done since the treatment of choice will vary

according to the severity of x, the patient's
age, the physician's skill, and the technology available at any given hospital. Moreover, there are some disorders for which
there is significant disagreement among
equally learned colleagues over what the
treatment of choice should be. Finally it is
not always clear that a patient has x since
there are any number of disorders with similar symptoms. Whatever may be the nature
and depth of his uncertainty, the physician
is usually forced by the patient's condition to
act before that uncertainty is resolved. In
this situation, the physician's action is dic-
tated by what he knows at the time. I am not
denying that there are diagnostic errors
made during the initial contact of physician
and patient and that some of these are sus-
tained until the patient's death. What I am
saying is that not all diagnoses and treatments that later experience proves wrong
are mistakes; some are actions that any
reasonable physician would have made under the circumstances. (23-24)

After reframing the question, four respondents downplayed risk-
factors while 11 acknowledged that untoward events do occur and
that risks are part of medical practice. I list typical responses below.
One nurse practitioner said:

There is the risk of life and limb in medicine.
All risks – litigation, loss of reputation – are
real. Early in my practice, I would do something, go home, and think about it. It would
keep me awake at night. I worked with a
colleague, however, who believed that the
kinds of cases that I see wouldn't kill someone. Yet, I still need to keep the risks in the
forefront of my work. You know that treating
colds and such cases aren't necessarily going to get you into trouble, but there are
things that I see as great risk – especially if I

misdiagnose or give a medication that is not
adequate to cover the problem. Potentially,
they could end up in the emergency room.
(Depicted as "11" in Table 5)

A physician said that even common illnesses can cause untoward
events. He said:

It's a reality of medicine for any family practitioner who is treating a cold that doesn't
get better. That's the nature of medicine.
Sometimes it doesn't work out.

Another claimed: "For me, untoward events are what I deal with
every day."

One respondent pointed out that physicians who practice procedures without understanding the behavioral patterns and environment of the patient are encouraging untoward events. Following
protocol may cure the symptom, but it may not solve the problem:

You have a male who is diabetic. His blood
sugars are all over the place. Now the
standard approach to this is education. The
assumption is that he does not know how to
handle his diabetes. He does not know how
to eat right or which exercise programs to
do. Therefore, a physician needs to tell him.
So, you're doing the medical model. This is
what is taught to physicians. But the reasons why a person's blood sugars are all
over the place is because, nine times out of
10, it is not due to not knowing, but rather it
is a matter of having some other need. Having to meet that need eliminates the ability
to control their diabetes. Let me give you an
example. We get people in their twenties
who come in and are in ketoacidosis. They
are real sick. Why? Because they don't
know? No! Because they are 21-year-old
people who, on Friday night, are sick and
tired of being diabetic. They want to go out
and eat pizza and drink beer. This is simply

because they are 21 years-old, and their
need is to be 21. This is a bigger need for
them than maintaining diabetes control. If
you don't understand that as well as deal
with them on that level, you are never going
to stop them from having recurrent ketoacidosis. So, to treat people, you have to work
within this lower level. (depicted as "13" in
Table 5)

Another respondent pointed out that physicians cannot treat patient
cases separate from the patients' environment and behaviors. That
respondent said:

We need to look at the big picture. So, if patients come in with a stress fracture, we can
work with them on why the stress fracture
occurred rather than just dealing with the
fracture by itself.

Another way that FP specialists fall into untoward events is by
misdiagnosing medical problems. One respondent states:

It's too easy to fall into a pattern of procedures and to forget to consider other variables that might explain what is happening to
the patient. So, it is possible that, when you
diagnose, you come to the wrong conclusion. Because you haven't considered some
other possibilities, you could actually start
applying the wrong procedure. Even though
you are following a correct protocol, you can
get into trouble. So learning how to look critically at types of problems in differential way
is extremely important. (depicted as "11" in
Table 5)

The first version of question three, namely, "Is the clinical practice of your specialty-interest area considered to be risky," tended
to elicit responses which can be categorized as denial of risk
(Thompson, 1993). These responses illustrate the belief that spe-

cialty-interest areas are non-risky. In Figure 8, I present this perspective "A". The horizontal line found half way down the funnel forms the divide between that perspective and another, quite different perspective (labeled as area "B" in Figure 8).

This second perspective is one where the practice of specialty-interest areas is viewed as risky because of the real possibility of the loss of life or limb, litigation, or loss of professional reputation.

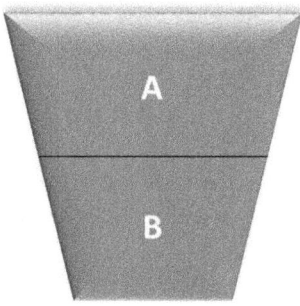

A = Denial of risks
B = Acknowledgements of risks

Figure 8. Perspectives Funnel

Question Four: How Did You Learn to Manage Untoward Events Associated with Doing Procedures in Your Specialty-Interest Area?

When procedures fail or when unforeseen events cause complications, untoward events occur. One way that FP specialists learn how to manage untoward events is to learn from models. One physician said:

> I worked with surgeons to learn what they do. They might teach me their diagnostic tricks so I can apply the tricks up front on someone.

Another stated:

> I learned from observing others in this field. I may engage in a discussion about, for example, their methodology in dealing with a type of problem.

One respondent stated that, by learning from other specialists builds confidence and competence in handling untoward events. She said:

> Some of it is trial-and-error, but much of it is learning from other physicians with whom I work. Even though I've been practicing since 1982, I really appreciate working with different people who practice and apply pearls. When I see their pearls, I'm amazed! Quite frankly, learning those pearls helped me become more independent. When I've been shown a pearl, I can go ahead and apply it the next time that problem comes up, and I know that it will probably work for me. (depicted as "10" in Table 5)

Another physician commented:

> I'm assuming that there are going to be some untoward events. So rather than simply trying to avoid them, it may be a matter of preparing myself for them. You learn to prepare for them when you first learn the procedure, when you have opportunities to discuss with colleagues on how they handle such cases and gather literature to support your understanding. (depicted as "4" in Table 4)

Some FP specialists rely on the combination of following protocols and luck for avoiding untoward events. One FP specialist said:

> One of the ways that we safeguard is by training ourselves to operate under protocol. If the problem does not fit the protocol, or if we just have a feeling about a case, we learn to get backup. (depicted as "1" in Table 3)

Another FP specialist explained that FP specialists need to recognize when a case, which normally can be handled routinely, gets out of control, and another when specialist must be called for help rather than trying to salvage the case alone. The FP specialist stated:

> In one case out of over a thousand vasectomies that I've done, I had to get help from a specialist. I called my urologist colleague and said: "I have a patient who is bleeding badly, and he is swelling to the size of a grapefruit. I need your help." The urologist came over, and we took the patient into surgery together. He found the artery causing the problem, and tied it. (depicted as "14" in Table 5)

Some physicians learned formal protocol for avoiding untoward events, which have been constructed and consensually established within the field. In sports medicine, one physician said that, due to the high risks, you must follow the national criteria to ensure safe play. Thus, the field has constructed some formal algorithms for handling untoward events. The physician said:

> This is typically not a negotiated issue. We must follow national criteria. For example, with a sprained ankle, there is no play until the player can show full range of motion and is able to jump 25 times on the effected ankle and run full speed with cutting. (depicted as "7" in Table 4)

Another physician gave a detailed description of how he learned to manage untoward events associated in doing procedures in his specialty-interest area. He stated:

> As I learned it, handling untoward events is best done when procedures and untoward events are considered together. When you're putting in a chest tube, you want to start lower than your entry point in the chest cavity between the two ribs when you go

through the skin. So the chest tube goes
through the skin up and over a rib, and then
between two ribs. When you pull the chest
tube out, that creates a seal. If you start out
right, you won't have a problem when you
take the chest tube out. You don't want to
go straight in, though, because that can create a sunken chest wound when you take
the tube out. You teach learners how to do
this by explaining that. You also must show
them how to avoid the nerve and artery,
which lie at the inferior border of each rib.
So they must understand to stay away from
the inferior border of each rib but, instead,
just work along the top of each rib and below it. (depicted as "8" in Table 5)

In contrast with this viewpoint, another FP specialist, whose interest area is acupuncture, believes that some types of problems
cannot be standardized. He said:

One of the complexities in acupuncture is
that there is no set point that you can use
for a particular condition. There may actually be different points. The other problem is
with standardization. Depending on which
approach you use, you might end up with a
different point for the same condition. In doing this, we categorize the kinds of problems, and then we must use strategies for
determining how to best approach that kind
of problem. (depicted as "6" in Table 4)

Another FP specialist learned to handle untoward events in another way. Because of the complexities of his specialty-interest area
and because no one was available to help him understand these
complexities, he entered another residency program to increase in
competence and confidence in handling this area. He stated:

When I first entered into this practice area, I
was very unclear about my roles, my duties,
and how to be responding to the laws and

regulations that are around that area. The question became: How does one do this ethically and intelligently? (depicted as "15" in Table 5)

Question Five: What Formal and Informal Support Networks Are Available in Your Specialty-Interest Area?

Respondents named national associations and, in some cases, national journals dedicated to specialty-interest areas. Geriatrics, sports medicine, acupuncture, occupational medicine, and emergency medicine have national organizations.

FP specialists also named informal support systems. All acknowledged colleagues for whom they might go to for mutual help and assistance. Some respondents noted, however, that it is possible, but not desirable, to practice a specialty-interest area on one's own, with little or no interaction with others in specialty-interest area.

Question Six: How Did You Learn Your Specialty-Interest Area?

Respondents reported that they learned their specialty-interest areas either by reception learning and autonomous learning, or they learned them by a form of cognitive apprenticeship. While no respondent reported learning by using guided inquiry or the Socratic method as their main mode of learning, this does not show that such learning didn't occur. It is possible that such types of learning supplemented reception learning. For example, respondent #1 (depicted as "1" and under "A" in Table 3) reported that reception learning occurred when a physician would review her patients' charts and tell her how to handle these cases. While I could classify the respondent's description as reception learning, it is possible that, on certain occasions, physicians complimented the reception learning by using other types of learning which they didn't report. What was reported, however, were the types of learning that the respondents considered to be the primary method.

Autonomous and Reception Learning

Nine of the interviewers reported that they learned their specialty-interest area through autonomous learning and reception learning. When using autonomous learning, FP specialists reported that they applied what they learned from family practice background to their specialty-interest area. Because the environmental conditions are different in a specialty-interest area (including working with athletes is different than working with lay patients due to different goals for recovery), FP specialists use trial-and-error to figure out what protocol best works for handling different types of problems. One physician said that helping workers on the job is much different than helping the typical patients in family practice. He stated, "No one was doing this type of work when I started. I had to figure it out for myself." A sports medicine physician expressed similar concerns when learning to work with athletes. He said:

> The way you learn how to work with athletes
> is by treating them. You need to figure out
> how to best meet their goal of getting back
> into play. You do this by practicing in the
> clinics. It's the best way. (depicted as "9" in
> Table 5)

Another FP specialist reported that she applied what she learned from psychology to help her patients with women's health issues. She stated:

> I have the personality for working with
> women and for helping them with their prob-
> lems. I brought into practice my interviewing
> skills and abilities to develop a rapport with
> patients. I've also had to apply what I've
> learned from my psychology classes in in-
> terviewing patients. (depicted as "3" in Table
> 4)

While autonomous learning can occur, FP specialists also use reception learning. FP specialists often supplement reception learning to improve practice rather than using autonomous learning alone. These reception-learning activities include reading guidelines for practicing within a specialty-interest area, seeking advice from other specialists, listening to or viewing tapes on how to handle specific types of cases, observing other specialists perform procedures, and reading journal articles.

One physician used reception learning to help him figure out how to apply FP protocol to occupational medicine. For him, he relied heavily on the notes from the previous physician, which were left at the industry plant, to understand how to deal with worker compensation problems.

A nurse practitioner learned on the job by observing models and listening to lectures. She said:

> I learned protocol from watching a fellow
> physician assistant perform procedures. I
> also spent time listening to guest lecturers
> on how they apply protocol.

FP specialists enrolled in courses to help them learn how to handle their specialty-interest areas. These respondents reported that these courses tended to be "lecture format" in which the FP specialists listened to experts in the field discuss how they handle case types. One FP specialist said, "The lectures helped me understand the principles used in geriatric medicine." Some reported that they enrolled in courses specifically designed to help FP specialists pass the certificate of added quality examinations. Such courses are also presented in a lecture format.

Cognitive Apprenticeship

Six respondents learned their specialty-interest area through forms of cognitive apprenticeship. Based on the data analyzed, none of the respondents reported learning their specialty-interest areas by using a pure form of cognitive apprenticeship. Moreover, all reported some form of reception learning which supplemented cognitive apprenticeship. For example, one respondent read about a procedure used by a physician in his specialty-interest area. Because the article didn't give enough information to perform the procedure, the respondent met with the physician, had the physician model how to use the procedure, practiced the procedure under the physician's supervision, and discussed how the procedure might vary if used in different types of cases.

All respondents using cognitive apprenticeship reported experiencing phases one and two. Phase one involved modeling as well as articulation of the principles, heuristics or tricks-of-the-trade to make them work, and pitfalls that can occur. Phase two involved practicing the procedure under scaffold conditions and with coaching. Based on the analysis of the data, I didn't find clear examples of phase three. Because learner focus is on the content of the learning and not on how they were being instructed, the respondents may not have recognized how trainers performed the fading.

One physician learned sports medicine by observing colleagues in the field and by working with other types of specialists. He observed surgeons modeling how to handle types of problems. He said:

> Before trying a procedure, the surgeons that
> I worked with would show me how they han-
> dle the ankle injury and would discuss with
> me what is involved in doing the procedure.

Another physician experienced reception learning as part of phase one. He reported:

> After listening to lectures and observing at-
> tendings demonstrating in clinics how to use
> the acupuncture points, I practiced in a lab
> setting under supervision.

A nurse practitioner reported that she learned how to perform differential diagnoses for types of rashes. She stated:

> The physician showed me how to differen-
> tially diagnose by looking at the appearance
> of a rash. He explained how to eliminate
> certain diagnoses and how to consider oth-
> ers as possibilities. He then explained ways
> that we might treat such rashes.

The nurse later reported, "The physician would check me out in the clinic to make sure I understood how to do the differential diagno-ses." This may be an example of phase three rather than phase two.

For phase four, respondents reported using trial-and-error to make the procedures work for them. What makes this different from autonomous learning is that these respondents were trained how to do procedures within the specialty-interest area rather than learning how to apply on their own procedures from family practice to the specialty-interest areas. For phase one through three, the respondents learned how to perform the procedure in an acceptable way (as constructed and consensually validated by the field). In phase four, the respondents learn how to perform the procedures in ways that work best for them.

One physician stated:

> When I tried this technique in my practice, I had to do some of this by trial-and-error, even though I was shown how to do it by my colleague at another university.

One physician learned how to check reflexes by taping on the bottom of the geriatric patient's foot rather than the kneecap. He found that this is less intrusive to the elderly patients.

Question Seven: How Do You Teach Others Your Specialty-Interest Area? If You Don't Teach it, How Would You Teach This Area to Another Specialist?

Five respondents reported using a wide variety of teaching methods. One stated, "I like to use the Socratic method during rounds. Of course, I would use this when time allowed." Another said:

> I find that all methods of learning except modeling without explanation are helpful.

One physician warned that autonomous learning can be deadly:

> When reading about a procedure in a journal article, all you're reading about is typically the principles involved. The researchers don't include the particulars of the procedures, such as what type of suture to use. Using the wrong one might cause trouble. What's dangerous is when someone tries to do a procedure without knowing the details. (depicted as "10" in Table 5)

Because one nurse practitioner had a successful practice, she trains others by using reception learning and autonomous learning. She said:

> I train nurses in the same way that I learned
> this field. By the time students work with
> me, they pretty much already know the pro-
> tocol. I tell them what they need to do and
> let them figure the rest out from there. They
> need to learn by practicing.

Ten teach or would teach using a form of cognitive apprentice-ship. A respondent stated:

> When you learn the procedures, we are
> taught the proper technique to do it. Varying
> in that technique can result in complications.
> To teach proper technique, you always
> demonstrate a procedure first. You show
> one, let them do one, and then they can
> teach one. When demonstrating, you ex-
> plain the procedure, how you can get in
> trouble, and what to do to avoid problems.
> (depicted as "8" in Table 5)

In working with limited time, one respondent said that there is only one effective way that he knows. He said:

> If we have only one night – a three-hour
> session – to teach a procedure. We start by
> defining the procedure, we show how it is
> done. We ask them to do it. Then, we cri-
> tique them.

Such training is a form of cognitive apprenticeship (Farmer, Buckmaster, and LeGrand, 1992; Brandt, Farmer, and Buckmaster, 1993).

Question Eight: How Has Family Practice Contributed to Your Specialty-Interest Area?

All respondents expressed that FP can influence specialty-interest areas in a unique way. FP specialists bring a holistic perspective that addresses more than the presenting problem. Other types of specialists may concern themselves with outlying factors but tend to focus only on the problem at hand. One respondent said:

> Family practice medicine provided me with breadth and basic foundations in medicine in a wide variety of areas, which is helpful in my going into a specialty interest.

Another respondent said:

> To be fair, there are other specialists that understand the larger dynamics, but family practice specialists are better trained in dealing with these issues and, consequently, do a better job.

In obstetrics, one physician claimed that dealing with the pregnancy separate from the patient's environment and behavioral problems can be a disservice. This respondent said:

> There is a lot more to helping a person than just simply preparing to deliver her baby. I'm the one who is going to work with her, when she is a mother, after I deliver her baby. For me, it is helpful to know what her home environment is like. Is she safe there? Does she have a support person? Sometimes you need to anticipate which ones are going to have difficulty raising their children, and which ones are going to be difficult to immunize. You might find out that she doesn't have a car or that her home life is volatile. You can almost predict who has more backaches and pelvic pain. You have to deal with the full-range of problems. (depicted as "4" in Table 4)

One physician claimed that you cannot go into a specialty-interest area with the mindset of a sub-specialist. You need to approach patients at the lower-end of the funnel as well as the upper-end (the funnel is depicted as Figure 8):

> I may be called a family-medicine purist. That means I believe in the concept of family medicine in its entirety. People do not exist in isolation. They exist in communities, be it family communities or the broader community. They exist in holistic manners and at multi-levels. You don't have patients who are pure bodies. (depicted as "9" in Table 5)

Question Nine: How Have Specialty-Interest Areas Contributed to Family Practice?

Respondents named two primary contributions that specialty-interest areas make in family practice. These are increased proficiencies in procedures and inner-departmental consultations.

First, FP specialists found that specialty-interest areas increase their understanding and skills of procedures. By focusing on an area, FP specialists better understand the more complex procedures involved in a specialty-interest area. A respondent who has a specialty interest in emergency medicine stated:

> Emergency care can help a physician become more skilled at doing a lot of procedures and in handling emergencies.

Another FP specialist said:

> What I found is that I now can better diagnose, for example, different grades of ankle sprain much better than when I just did family practice. Those in this area taught me how to handle ankle sprains in a much different and better way. (depicted as "7" in Table 4)

A physician, whose area is sports medicine, said that he can now handle muscular-skeletal illnesses and injuries better as well as sports-related ones. He said, "Such injuries can include, for example, a 45-year-old man who decides to take up running and injures himself."

Another way that specialty-interest areas contribute to family practice is in consultation and education. As FP specialists become known for having incorporated a specialty-interest area in their practices, other physicians may refer patients to them or consult with them about cases. One stated:

> My colleagues know that I have this interest, so I tend to receive more cases in my family practice. Often times, my colleagues will consult with me in the office if they have a particular case in this area. They might say: "Can you look at this x-ray or how would you handle this? (depicted as "9" in Table 5)

Another said:

> Not only are my skills in dealing with these things better utilized in my practice, but my opinions and judgements are also sought out. People in the clinics will request for me to suture this wound, put this cast on, treat this fracture, or look at this x-ray. (depicted as "8" in Table 5)

Specialty-interest areas offer opportunities for educating colleagues. One physician stated that this was an important role for a FP unit. He described collegial support as an important part of continuing education. He said:

> If you have an office where doctors have different interest areas, they can ask each other questions and learn from each other. I think that this educational process works extremely well.

Three Distinct Patterns of Relationship

From my data analysis, I identified three distinct patterns (referred to as "ways") of relationships between responses to the interview questions. I depict the three ways in figures 9, 10, and 11. Each way is grounded in how respondents view the level of risks involved in practicing within specialty-interest areas. Moreover, each way describes how respondents learned their current practice in their specialty-interest area and how the teach or would teach their specialty-interest area to other specialists.

Way 1: Specialty-Interest Areas as Relatively Safe

One respondent reported that the practice in specialty-interest areas is relatively safe, which is depicted as Figure 9.

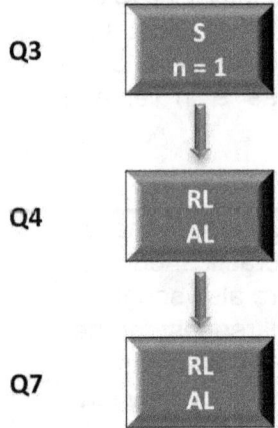

Q3 = Can untoward events occur?
Q4 = How did you learn your specialty-interest area?
Q7 = How do you (or would you) teach your specialty-interest area?
S = No untoward events occur and field is relatively safe
RL = Reception learning
AL = Autonomous learning

Figure 9. FP Specialists that View Specialty-Interest Areas as Relatively
        Safe

FP specialists who view specialty-interest areas from this perspective learned their specialty-interest area by reception learning and autonomous learning. The respondent likewise instructs using the same types of learning.

Way 2: Specialty-Interest Area as Somewhat Safe

Six respondents reported that practicing in specialty-interest areas is somewhat safe. This is depicted as Figure 10.

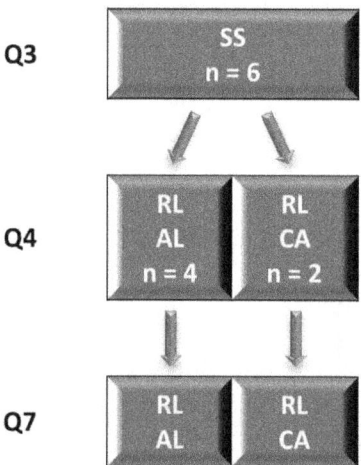

Q3 = Can untoward events occur?
Q4 = How did you learn your specialty-interest area?
Q7 = How do you (or would you) teach your specialty-interest area?
SS = Untoward events can occur, but the field is somewhat safe
RL = Reception learning
AL = Autonomous learning
CA = Cognitive apprenticeship

Figure 10. FP Specialists that View Specialty-Interest Areas
        as Somewhat Safe

While procedures may be performed to handle most medical cases, untoward events can occur. However, by learning medical procedures along with some basic risk management procedures, these FP specialists believe that medical cases can be controlled and managed with little risk occurring. One FP specialist, who sees sports medicine as somewhat safe, stated that there are strict national criteria that must be followed to ensure the safety of players in sports medicine. The same FP specialist also said, "I find that all methods of learning except modeling without explanation are useful."

Some learned by using autonomous and reception learning. Others learned from a combination of reception learning and a form of cognitive apprenticeship. Consequently, those in this group instruct the way that they learned their specialty-interest area.

Way 3: Specialty-Interest Area as Risky

Those who follow way three view the field as being risky. This is depicted as Figure 11. While some learned by reception learning and autonomous learning, others learned by reception learning and forms of cognitive apprenticeship. Both, however, teach or would teach using forms of cognitive apprenticeship supplemented with reception learning.

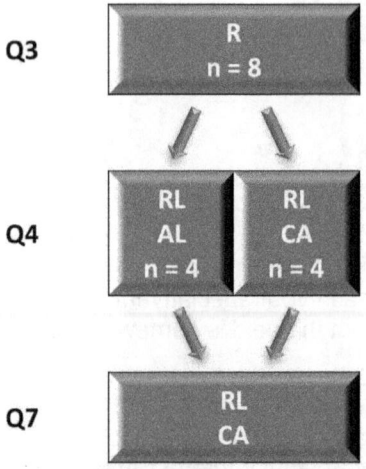

Q3 = Can untoward events occur?
Q4 = How did you learn your specialty-interest area?
Q7 = How do you (or would you) teach your specialty-interest area?
R   = Untoward events can occur, and the field is risky
RL = Reception learning
AL = Autonomous learning
CA = Cognitive apprenticeship

Figure 11. FP Specialists that View Specialty-Interest Areas as Risky

Function	Respondent 1	
	A	B
Modeling	X	X
Articulation of Principles, Tricks, and Risk Management	X	X
Coaching	?	?
Scaffolding	X	X
Fading	X	X
Internalization	X	X
Generalization	X	X
Feedback	✓	✓
Invention	✓	✓
Observing	✓	✓
Reading	✓	✓
Listening	✓	✓
Socratic Dialogue	?	?
Talking through a Procedure	✓	✓
Hands-on Training	✓	✓
Trial-and-Error	✓	✓

Column A = Respondent's learning a specialty-interest area
Column B = Respondent's instructing a specialty-interest area
X   = Function not used by respondent
✓   = Function used by respondent
?   = Research is unclear if respondent experienced function

Table 3. Way 1: Functions Involved in Learning and Instructing

Function	Respondents											
	2		3		4		5		6		7	
	A	B	A	B	A	B	A	B	A	B	A	B
Modeling	X	X	X	X	X	X	X	X	✓	✓	✓	✓
Articulation of Principles, Tricks, and Risk Management	X	X	X	X	X	X	X	X	✓	✓	✓	✓
Coaching	X	X	X	X	?	?	?	?	✓	✓	✓	✓
Scaffolding	X	X	X	X	X	X	X	X	✓	✓	?	✓
Fading	X	X	X	X	X	X	X	X	?	?	?	?
Internalization	X	X	X	X	X	X	X	X	?	?	?	?
Generalization	X	X	X	X	X	X	X	X	✓	?	?	?
Invention	✓	✓	✓	✓	✓	✓	✓	✓	X	X	X	X
Observing	✓	✓	✓	✓	✓	✓	✓	✓	✓	✓	✓	✓
Reading	✓	✓	✓	✓	✓	✓	✓	✓	✓	✓	✓	✓
Listening	✓	✓	✓	✓	✓	✓	✓	✓	✓	✓	✓	✓
Socratic Dialogue	?	?	?	?	?	?	?	✓	?	?	?	?
Talking through a Procedure	✓	✓	✓	✓	✓	✓	✓	✓	✓	✓	✓	✓
Hands-on Training	✓	✓	✓	✓	✓	✓	✓	✓	✓	✓	✓	✓
Trial-and-Error	✓	✓	✓	✓	✓	✓	✓	✓	?	?	?	?

Column A = Respondent's learning a specialty-interest area
Column B = Respondent's instructing a specialty-interest area
X = Function not used by respondent
✓ = Function used by respondent
? = Research is unclear if respondent experienced function

Table 4. Way 2: Functions Involved in Learning and Instructing

Function	Respondents							
	8		9		10		11	
	A	B	A	B	A	B	A	B
Modeling	✓	✓	X	✓	✓	✓	✓	✓
Articulation of Principles, Tricks, and Risk Management	✓	✓	X	✓	✓	✓	✓	✓
Coaching	✓	✓	X	✓	✓	✓	✓	✓
Scaffolding	✓	✓	X	?	✓	✓	?	?
Fading	?	✓	X	?	?	?	?	✓
Internalization	?	?	X	?	✓	?	✓	✓
Generalization	?	✓	X	?	?	?	?	?
Invention	X	X	X	X	X	X	X	X
Observing	✓	✓	✓	✓	✓	✓	✓	✓
Reading	✓	✓	✓	✓	✓	✓	✓	✓
Listening	✓	✓	✓	✓	✓	✓	✓	✓
Socratic Dialogue	?	?	?	?	?	?	?	?
Talking through a Procedure	✓	✓	✓	✓	✓	✓	✓	✓
Hands-on Training	✓	✓	✓	✓	✓	✓	✓	✓
Trial-and-Error	?	?	?	?	?	?	?	?

Column A = Respondent's learning a specialty-interest area
Column B = Respondent's instructing a specialty-interest area
  X   = Function not used by respondent
  ✓   = Function used by respondent
  ?   = Research is unclear if respondent experienced function

Table 5. Way 3: Functions Involved in Learning and Instructing

[table continues]

[table 5 continued]

Function	Respondents							
	12		13		14		15	
	A	B	A	B	A	B	A	B
Modeling	X	✓	X	✓	X	✓	✓	✓
Articulation of Principles, Tricks, and Risk Management	X	✓	X	✓	X	✓	✓	✓
Coaching	X	✓	X	✓	X	✓	✓	✓
Scaffolding	X	✓	X	✓	X	✓	✓	✓
Fading	X	?	X	?	?	?	?	?
Internalization	X	?	X	?	X	?	✓	?
Generalization	X	?	X	✓	?	?	?	?
Invention	✓	?	✓	✓	✓	✓	X	X
Observing	X	✓	?	?	✓	✓	✓	✓
Reading	✓	✓	✓	✓	✓	✓	✓	✓
Listening	X	✓	✓	✓	✓	✓	✓	✓
Socratic Dialogue	?	?	?	?	?	?	?	?
Talking through a Procedure	✓	✓	✓	✓	✓	✓	✓	✓
Hands-on Training	✓	✓	✓	✓	✓	✓	✓	✓
Trial-and-Error	?	?	?	?	?	?	?	?

Column A = Respondent's learning a specialty-interest area
Column B = Respondent's instructing a specialty-interest area
　X　　 = Function not used by respondent
　✓　　 = Function used by respondent
　?　　 = Research is unclear if respondent experienced function

Table 5 [continued]. Way 3: Functions Involved in Learning and Instructing

Evidence from the Findings of the Issue Facing FP Specialists Who Developed Specialty-Interest Areas

From my analysis shown in Figures 9, 10, and 11, I discovered three issues with developing specialty-interest areas.

First, I found that respondents struggled between having to invent procedures and being socialized to acceptable practices. Later, I describe this as struggling with the horns of a learning dilemma.

Second, I found that respondents developed their specialty-interest areas through autonomous and reception learning but train or would train others using social-cognitive learning.

Third, I found evidence of three patterns of learning or instructing for developing specialty-interest areas. The three ways associate with viewing the practice of specialty-interest areas as being safe, somewhat safe, or risky.

Summary

In this chapter, I presented my data collection findings. I described the respondents, key informants, survey questionnaire findings, one-on-one interview findings, three distinct patterns of learning, summary of the types of learning, and evidence of the issues facing FP specialists who have developed specialty-interest areas.

Chapter 6

Discussion: Resolving the Three-Way Interlocking Dilemma

From the interviews, I identified three patterns or ways of learning and instructing FP specialists who want to develop specialty-interest areas. I also found evidence of FP specialists who learned their specialty-interest areas by autonomous and reception learning but when instructing others (or when considering how they would instruct others), they would use social-cognitive learning. Lastly, I found a complex, three-way interlocking dilemma.

In this chapter, I discuss these findings and how to answer the research question:

> What type(s) of learning best explain how
> FP specialists engage in specialty-interest
> areas without becoming another type of
> specialist?

The Three-Way Interlocking Dilemma

From my analysis, I found a complex dilemma. This dilemma makes the process of expanding from family medicine to specialty-interest areas to be puzzling and potentially problematic. The complex dilemma consists of three separate but interrelated dilemmas, as depicted as Figure 12. The three-way interlocking dilemmas are:

- Control vs. autonomy
- Procedure vs. invention
- Safe practice vs. risky practice

These dilemmas are complexly interrelated because FP specialists can become entangled in them in different ways, depending on the circumstances of the situation. Different environmental factors, personal factors, and behavioral factors may influence how FP specialists become caught in the dilemma.

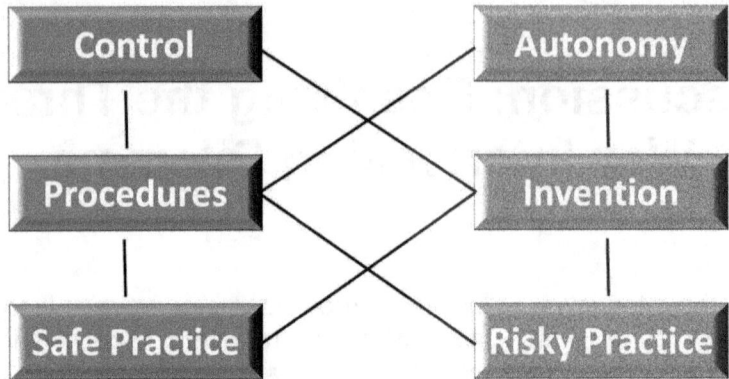

Figure 12. The Three-Way Interlocking Dilemma

For example, in one circumstance, FP specialists:

- View their practice as being safe (safe-practice horn)
- Select a known routine from family practice (procedure horn)
- Try to figure out on their own how to make that routine work with patients within the specialty-interest area (autonomy horn)

In another circumstance, those same FP specialists:

- View a situation as potentially problematic (risky horn)
- Use protocol learned in family medicine (procedure horn)
- Perform the protocol under the close supervision of a FP specialist in the specialty-interest area (control horn)

In a third circumstance, the same FP specialists:

- View their work as safe (safe horn)
- Try to make up a procedure for handling an unusual ill-defined case (invention horn)

- Figure out how to make the new procedure work with this and other similar cases (autonomy horn)

I illustrate these three circumstances in Figure 13.

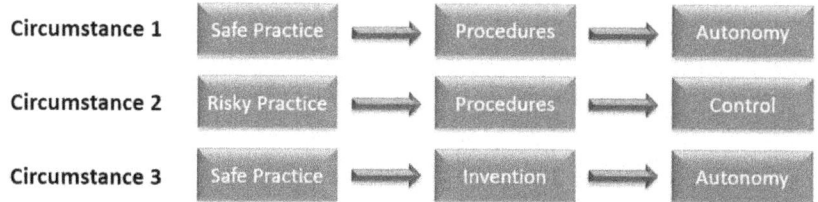

Figure 13. FP specialists can shift horns given different circumstances

To mitigate confusion and problematic thinking, FP specialists need to resolve this complex dilemma. Before I discuss the specific dilemmas involved in developing specialty-interest areas and how FP specialists can reframe them, in the next section, I explain how Petrie (1991) and Kemmel (1980) comprehend dilemmas. Their models give a structure for discussing the characteristics of dilemmas that FP specialists encounter when developing specialty-interest areas as part of their practice. These models also offer insight into the various conditions and constraints that can affect how FP specialists resolve dilemmas.

Two Approaches for Resolving Dilemmas

Introduction

In this section, I present Petrie's (1991) approach for resolving dilemmas and Kimmel's (1980) approach. Each model:

- Explains characteristics of dilemmas
- Describes two horns of dilemmas
- Portrays the process for handling dilemmas
- Explains the emergent value

Petrie's Approach to Resolving Dilemmas

Horns of a Dilemma

Dilemmas consist of two conflicting or opposing viewpoints,

tendencies, perspectives, methods of operation, or philosophical approaches (Petrie, 1991). Petrie metaphorically describes the diametric viewpoints as horns of a dilemma. Each horn offers insight into how FP specialists function within their field. FP specialists can benefit by accepting one horn and even prosper. Yet, each horn has weaknesses as well as strengths. While FP specialists can gain insight by pursuing one horn, the horn causes some biases. Blinded by such biases, negative consequences can occur unexpectedly.

Consider this example: Assume that there is a dilemma between patient advocacy and complying with strict worker compensation laws within occupational medicine (two horns of the dilemma). Susan, a new FP physician, has been trained in family medicine to promote the wants and needs of patients (the patient-advocacy horn). In an occupational setting, Susan may inadvertently cause negative consequences by over-emphasizing the patient-advocacy horn. Management offices could cause tension by complaining that Susan isn't getting patients back to work promptly. Patients may become depressed because Susan keeps them on worker compensation too long. Susan might even face litigation if she doesn't comply with worker compensation laws. If Susan only engages in strict compliance, she may experience a different set of negative consequences. Workers may become injured due to having to return to work prematurely, and workers may pursue litigation against Susan for not protecting them.

FP specialists can experience dilemmas in one of four behaviors. First, FP specialists may not understand the broad scope of their environment. Without realizing the full range of options, they may unconsciously be taken in and *hooked* by one horn. While a horn may be appealing for managing well-defined situations, FP specialists may be caught off guard by ill-defined, unfavorable, or risky conditions that the horn doesn't account for.

The second behavior is when FP specialists recognize that there are two opposing perspectives or horns and are unable to resolve the conflicting views.

The third behavior occurs when FP specialists resolve the dilemma immediately but without realizing that a dilemma existed.

With the fourth behavior, FP specialists identify the dilemma, struggle with it, and then resolve it. I discuss resolving dilemmas in the next section.

Resolving Dilemmas

FP specialists may become seduced by one horn of a dilemma. They grasp the horn to the exclusion of the other one, and they become hooked by it. To overcome a dilemma effectively, Petrie (1991) states that FP specialists must understand the strengths of the two horns while acknowledging the weaknesses. They must then shift to an adaptive process in which they struggle with the two horns using assimilation and accommodation. Without excluding one or the other horn, they must reflect upon how to integrate both horns. Petrie describes this process as slipping between the horns of dilemma.

In the earlier example, Susan struggled between promoting patient advocacy and complying with strict worker compensation laws within occupational medicine. Both horns offer insight into quality of care, but both have pitfalls and weaknesses. By reflecting upon each horn, Susan can identify situations in which patient advocacy is necessary while being aware of compliance. By struggling with both extremes, Susan can develop a new philosophical approach for working within occupational medicine.

Kimmel's Approach to Resolving Dilemmas

Like Petrie, Kimmel (1980) discusses dilemmas and how to resolve them. Kimmel draws heavily from Erikson's (1976) approach. In his Kimmel's model, dilemmas have two opposing tendencies. These tendencies cause a dialectical struggle in which those forced with a dilemma are attracted to both but cannot accept fully one over the other. By reframing the approach to accepting both tendencies instead of rejecting one, FP specialists can overcome the dilemma.

Kimmel advocate the following steps for resolving dilemmas:

1. Recognize the two choices of the dilemma in which both are attractive and beneficial.
2. Acknowledge that accepting one alternative and rejecting the other can lead to undesirable consequences.
3. Decide which of the two horns should be situationally considered the more favorable one. The favorable one is the syntonic choice, and the less favorable one is the dystonic choice. The syntonic must absorb but not destroy the dystonic one for an emergent value to occur.

The Dilemma of Control and Autonomy

Introduction

One of the dilemmas facing FP specialists who developed specialty-interest areas is the autonomy vs. control dilemma. In this section, I explain each horn characteristics along with the emergent value that FP specialists can experience by resolving the dilemma.

Characteristics of the Two Horns of the Autonomy/Control Dilemma

The Horn of Autonomy

FP specialists who are caught on the horn of autonomy subscribe to the following belief: Entering a specialty-interest area entails only applying the principles, risk management, and heuristics or tricks-of-the-trade learned from the FP field to the specialty-interest area setting. Because FP specialists have had some initial experience in most specialty-interest areas while in residency (such as sports medicine, geriatrics, obstetrics, and adolescent medicine), they may assume that figuring out how to apply principles, protocols, and routines is a simple task. Furthermore, they assume that this is a low-risk practice. Having a medical foundation in family practice is enough to overcome any pitfalls because their profession has already identified such pitfalls. Moreover, socializing new FP specialists to a specialty-interest area involves no real risks.

Those who subscribe to this horn fall into one of two categories. First, it may be the case that the FP specialists have not truly entered a specialty-interest area, and so they are still practicing within the traditional scope of family practice. Thus, there is no difference between how they function in this area and how other FP specialists function who do not claim to have engaged in a specialty-interest area. Therefore, such individuals are practicing from the gold standards of family practice. No further socialization to the chosen specialty-interest area has occurred.

The second possibility is that the FP specialists have entered a specialty-interest area (depicted as "A" in Figure 14) but have not been socialized to that specialty-interest area.

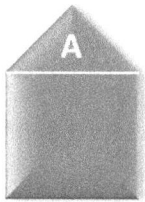

A = FP specialists who invent and innovate ways to apply procedures from FP to their specialty-interest areas

Figure 14. The First Piece of the Puzzle: The Tip of the Iceberg or the Horn of Autonomy

Instead of having another FP specialist who has developed the specialty-interest areas successfully to articulate how to best apply procedures to that specialty-interest area, they become overly optimistic in their abilities to successfully apply FP principles, risk management, and heuristics or tricks-of-the-trade to the specialty-interest area. They also overestimate their ability to handle problems by denying or ignoring the high-risk nature of all medicine. In the findings chapter, one respondent reflected this. She said:

> I worked with a colleague who believed that
> the kinds of cases that I see wouldn't kill
> someone.

Another said, "I try not to think about possible risks." Respondents who grasp this horn express that they can successfully figure out ways of applying procedures through trial-and-error, innovation, invention or experimentation, which prevents their work from becoming risky. By using innovative and creative applications of FP procedures, respondents believe that they can control for pitfalls and untoward events, thus making their work relatively safe or somewhat safe.

The error of being seduced by this horn hits hardest when FP specialists try to apply principles, routines, and protocols that fail. As noted in the chapter 3, one physician, who initially chose this approach but found it strenuous, said, "It was baptism by fire." When another physician entered his specialty-interest area, he found that the procedures of patient advocacy conflicted with the legal demands of worker compensation and with the demands of industrial management. Once the tensions and problems of applying FP principles became desperate, the physician chose to enter a second residency to learn how to accurately practice medicine in this new arena.

Trying to figure out the application of FP procedures in a particular setting can result in untoward events, such as:

- Loss of life and limb
- Emotional distress to patients and family
- Litigation
- Loss of professional reputation

Even when this happens, FP specialists who are hooked on the autonomy horn might deny responsibility or may rationalize what occurred.

Horn of Control

FP specialists who subscribe to this viewpoint recognize that FP specialists cannot simply apply the gold standards of family practice directly to specialty-interest areas. Rather, socialization is needed to help new FP specialists understand difference in philosophy, environmental concerns, and new ways of applying procedures. As exemplified in chapter 3, one physician said that he learned a different approach to handling sprains within the specialty-interest area of sports medicine. This approach was specifically designed to help athletes return to their sport within a short period, while the family practice approach is designed to ensure that the injury is completely healed before returning to normal activities. Thus, the FP approach is inadequate to serve the needs of athletes due to inefficiencies in addressing the full range of the patients' concerns. This approach assumes that specialty-interest areas offer a different way of practicing medicine, and it suggests that FP specialists need to be socialized to practice specialty-interest areas and avoid the applicative fallacy.

Those attracted to the horn of control recognize that the type of practice that they do is not completely safe. Within specialty-interest areas, pitfalls and untoward events exists and need to be handled when they occur. FP specialists believe that the way to handle such problems is to socialize FP specialists to the gold standards of the specialty-interest area. In chapter 3, for example, one respondent said, "The protocol protects us." Thus, the socialization process to the procedures and risk management prevent untoward events.

While the horn of autonomy encourages FP specialists to invent, innovate, use trial-and-error practice, and experiment to develop their own procedures, the horn of control encourages FP specialists to conform to well-defined procedures. This encouragement can lead to an over-reliance of procedures.

Much of FP socialization (depicted as "A" in Figure 15) does manage to control for potential untoward events, but these FP specialists must rely on basic risk management skills, good luck, and the possibility that another specialist might need to bail them out in case of an untoward event (depicted as "B" in Figure 15).

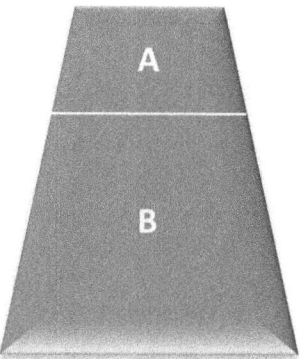

A = Routine procedures being handled from the perspective of FP
B = Risk management procedures for handling untoward events from the perspective of FP

Figure 15. The Tip and Main Body of the Iceberg: The Horn of Control

In chapter 3, one respondent said:

> One of the ways that we safeguard is by training ourselves to operate under protocol. If the problem does not fit the protocol, or if you just have a feeling about a case, I learned to get backup.

Because of the over-dependence on procedures, two serious negative consequences could occur:

First, FP specialists may have a medical case that cannot be handled by standard procedure, but they may still inaccurately perceive that they can handle the problem using standard protocol. Per Petrie (1991), professionals may see what they want to see, namely that they can handle the medical case with procedures instead of recognizing the case to be anomalous. Therefore, FP specialists may believe that they can handle the problem but end up over extending the effectiveness of the procedure. They lack the ability to handle such problems resulting in disaster.

The second way that FP specialists can experience negative consequences is by extensively relying on other specialists to handle atypical problems. If they do not learn to manage pitfalls and untoward events, FP specialists may refer too quickly to other types of specialists. If this often happens, organizational expenses increase under a capitated system due to the higher number of expensive and unnecessary referrals to other specialists.

Resolving the Autonomy/Control Dilemma

Overview

For FP specialists to resolve the autonomy/control dilemma, they must accept both horns in a particular, integrated approach. Neither horn can be completely rejected, for both offer substantial benefits for practice. FP specialists need to consider the control horn to be the syntonic – the more favorable – and to consider the autonomy horn to be dystonic – the less favorable. Because FP specialists remain within the field of family practice rather than become another type of specialist, their primary field continues to exert extensive control while the specialty-interest area that they developed exerts additional control. Relevant specialties, such as orthopaedic surgery for sports medicine and obstetrics/gynecology for obstetrics, also exert control. Rather than practicing the specialty-interest area autonomously, FP specialists enter work under the control of these fields. At the same time, FP specialists cannot afford to practice procedures rigidly or in a rote manner if they are to function effectively as FP specialists in their specialty-interest area. Functioning under control but with flexibility is what Thompson (1993) refers to as *bounded flexibility*.

Assimilation and Accommodation

By resolving the autonomy/control dilemma, FP specialists develop an emergent value: bounded flexibility. Bounded flexibility involves adapting a reflective equilibrium between assimilation and accom-

modation (Petrie, 1991). As depicted in Figure 16, this adaption resolves the dilemma. To be adaptive, FP specialists assimilate the
control horn while accommodating the autonomous horn.

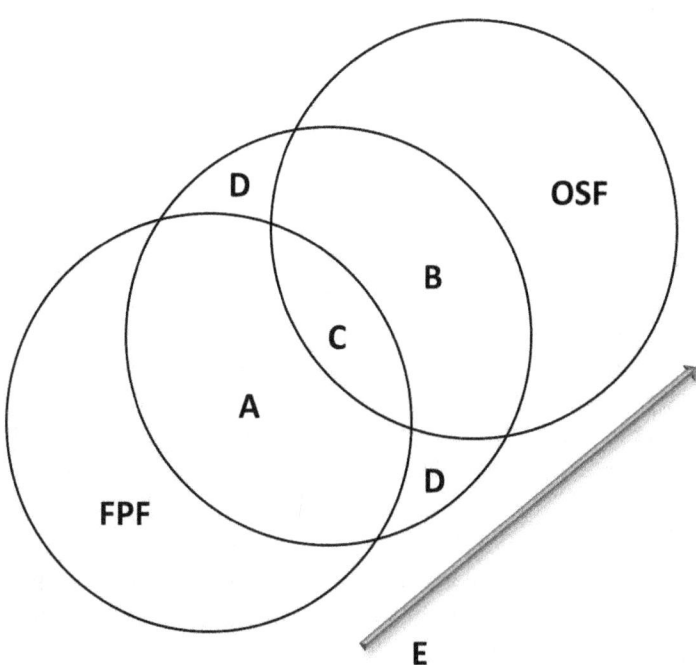

FPF = FP field
OSF = Other specialty field
A   = Assimilating procedures from FP to specialty-interest areas
B   = Accommodating procedures from relevant other specialty fields
       to specialty-interest areas
C   = Procedures that are common between FP and other relevant
       specialty areas
D   = Procedures unique to specialty-interest areas
E   = Direction of development for FP specialists entering a specialty-
       interest area

Figure 16. Relation of FP, Specialty-Interest Areas, and Other Special-
          ties

Assimilation

Assimilation is the part of adaptiveness in which learners socialize to how FP protocols and routines apply to the specialty-interest area. Assimilation occurs because the conceptual schemes of the field, which Petrie (1991) calls *norm-regarding behavior*, do not radically change. This includes internalizing the procedures so that they work well for the FP specialists (such as what happens during the internalization phase of cognitive apprenticeship).

Assimilation enables FP specialists to unify, classify, and standardize the wide range of medical cases which often occurs in practice. By using norms in medical practice, specialists can rationally "access our perceptions, behaviors, and beliefs." (Petrie, 1991, 118). Doing so enables specialists to manage and control responsibly. For example, Sam, a FP specialist, enters occupational medicine and serves a new set of clients from an industrial factory. Sam may need to assimilate family medicine protocols and routines to meet the unique needs of workers, factory owners, and society.

Accommodation

Assimilation is only one part of the strategy for adaptiveness. When norms and rules do not aid in assimilating an experience, accommodation is necessary.

Failure to assimilate can be due to two reasons. First, a particular medical case differs from the guiding norm such as when an environmental change makes the norm ineffective. This variation could be a constructive or destructive bug. For example, a community becomes ill due to polluted drinking water.

The second possibility is that FP specialists expect too much from the guiding norm (an internal perception). This fallacy relates to the control horn: those who are hooked by the control horn believe that socializing to protocols and routines is enough to protect FP specialists from untoward events. This fallacy is exemplified when FP specialists falsely believe that the norms, which they are familiar with, apply to all types of fractures when, in fact, this is not the case. Because environments where types of fractures can occur may vary and because the patients' physical characteristics can differ, norms cannot capture the full range of variation.

Per Petrie (1991), disturbances and puzzles, which are different from typical problems, tend to resist the ordinary applications of the norms. When these disturbances persist and specialists cannot assimilate to them, Petrie considers such puzzles to be anomalies. At this point, a crisis stage occurs. If specialists cannot find a reasonable alternative approach, then the anomalies are classified as destructive bugs. If an alternative way reframes the puzzle so that it no longer is a disturbance, then accommodation occurs. FP specialists who developed specialty-interest areas use accommodation (depicted as "B" in Figure 16) when they incur situations which they cannot handle using procedures that the FP field has constructed and consensually validated. Instead, FP specialists adapt another field's procedures in which that field constructed and consensually validated for use by FP specialists who entered specialty-interest areas. In other words, FP specialists are practicing procedures uniquely as part of the cadre of FP specialists who entered that specialty-interest area rather than behaving as freelance, individualistic problem solvers or as if they were specialists from another field.

Limitations in Resolving the Control/Autonomy Dilemma

The control/autonomy issue is a psychological and an administrative way to understand the complex dilemma. Resolution of the control/autonomy dilemma only indicates the emergent value, bounded flexibility (Thompson, 1993). Thompson gives little to no guidance about how to operationalize bounded flexibility. To do so, one must grasp both the safe and risk horns of the safety/risk dilemma. When you consider the risk horn to be the syntonic and the safe horn to be the dystonic and the syntonic absorbs but doesn't destroy the dystonic, what results is analogous to bounded flexibility and is referred to in the literature as internalization (Vygotsky, 1992). This is achieved when cognitive apprenticeship is successful in socializing specialists to handle certain types of situations using procedures that have been constructed and consensually validated by the profession in ways that work well for them and ways that are situationally appropriate within the bounds that are acceptable to the field and society.

The Safe/Risk Dilemma

The safe/risk dilemma appears to be the key to the complex dilemma. The safe/risk dilemma refines and elaborates on the three ways for developing specialty-interest areas, as described by respondents in this study, depicted in Figures 9, 10, and 11 in chapter 3. I present each way considering the safe/risk dilemma.

Way 1: Specialty-Interest Areas as Relatively Safe

Those FP specialists who follow the first way assume that the field is relatively safe, as depicted in Figure 17.

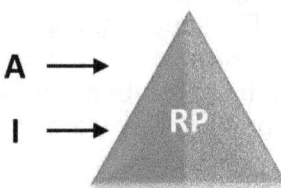

A   = Applying what was learned from FP
B   = Inventing how to apply what was learned from FP
RP = Routines and procedures

Figure 17. Specialty-Interest Areas Are Perceived as Being Safe: The First Way of Interpreting How FP Specialists Enter Specialty-Interest Areas

FP specialists perceive that they can handle routinely most the case types. Much of their work involves performing the proper protocol and routines for any given situation. By successfully following protocol and routines, FP specialists should avoid difficulties. From this viewpoint, FP specialists can learn procedures using any type of learning, especially reception learning and autonomous learning.

While perceiving medicine in this way offers a sense of control, this approach denies that underlying risks can occur. Like the tip of an iceberg, however, FP specialists who subscribes to way one fail to perceive the dangers that lie below.

Here are three reasons why a FP specialist might subscribe to way one:

1. The schema from how specialists were trained in the FP field and the schema of how to practice medicine can powerfully effect how they understand and engage in practice and learning. FP specialists might perceive developing specialty-interest areas by applying the FP schema to that new area.
2. There is a general tendency for over-optimism and over-belief of control in high risk fields, per Thompson (1993).
3. How instructors instructed FP specialists in medical school could dispose them to use a behavioral approach to learning.

Way 2: Specialty-Interest Areas as Somewhat Safe

FP specialists may perceive specialty-interest areas by a second way in which they consider the practice to be somewhat safe, as depicted as Figure 18. While they consider that much of medical practice to be routine, they recognize that untoward events can

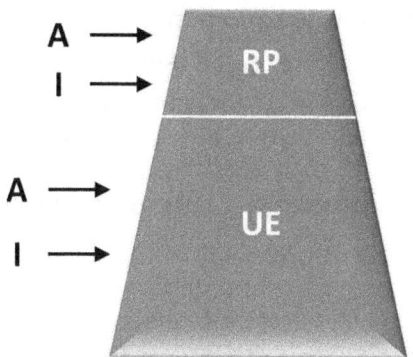

A   = Applying what was learned from FP
B   = Inventing how to apply what was learned from FP
RP = Routines and procedures
UE = Untoward Events

Figure 18. Somewhat Safe: The Second Way of Interpreting How FP Specialists Enter Specialty-Interest Areas

occur. FP Specialists who acknowledge this believe that the procedures for handling pitfalls can protect them from untoward events. These FP specialists might rely some on luck and the possibility of another type of specialist or similar specialist can help them recover or rescue them from untoward events. They tend to apply what they learned from the FP field and innovate some to learn how to handle both routine situations and untoward events.

Way 3: Specialty-Interest Areas as Risky

While the first two ways perceive specialty-interest areas as being relatively safe or somewhat safe, FP specialists who follow the third way perceive specialty-interest areas as risky, as depicted in Figure 19. In contrast to the first two ways in which FP specialists focus on developing individualistic problem-solving skills, the third way focuses on socializing FP specialists to function proficiently in area "A", "B", "C", and "D" in Figure 16.

In Figure 19, the upward arrow, "A", represents the perspective taken when FP specialists view their work as being risky. FP specialists recognize that the specialty-interest areas have constructed and consensually validated ways on how FP specialists handle rescue responsibly. In way three, no procedures are taught without instructing how to handle associated untoward events at the same time. Learning to handle both must be considered when determining the zone of proximal development of learners.

The downward arrow, "B", represents socialization to whole and fragmented procedures that the specialty-interest areas fields have constructed and consensually validated for handling types of situations. Area one, "RP", represents the most frequent types of problems in which FP specialists can handle using procedures.

"R1" depicts untoward events that can occur due to error in performing procedures and external pitfalls in which the specialty-interest area fields codified rescue procedures that the field has constructed and consensually validated. "R2" represents types of untoward events for which the field constructed and consensually validated fragments (such as heuristics or tricks-of-the-trade) for rescue. Even though only fragmented forms exist, these are better than using a trial-and-error, individualistic approach.

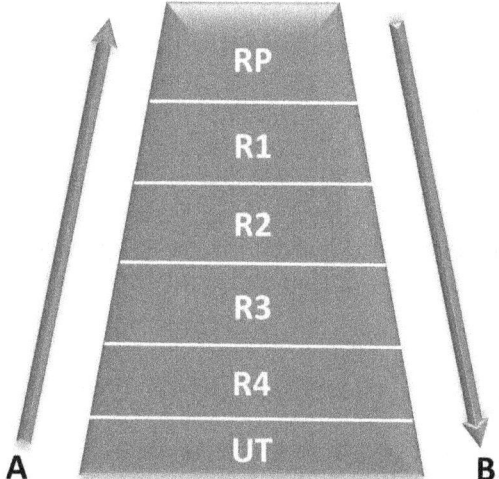

A   = Perspective taken when the work is viewed as risky
B   = Socialization to the whole and fragmented procedures
RP = Routines and procedures
R1 = Whole, codified rescue procedures
R2 = Codified fragments of rescue procedures
R3 = Whole, codified compromised rescue
R4 = Codifed fragments for compromised rescue
UT = Unknown territory

Figure 19. Risky: The Third Way of Examining How FP Specialists Enter Specialty-Interest Areas

"R3" and "R4" represent untoward events in which rescue without compromising the patient's health cannot occur. Therefore, the goal shifts to salvaging the situation as best as one can. In "R3", untoward events occur in which uncompromised results cannot be achieved. The specialty-interest areas field has constructed and consensually validated whole, codified compromised rescue procedures, and experts can train FP specialists to appropriately use them. In "R4", there are only codified fragments (such as heuristics or tricks-of-the-trade) for FP specialists to use in compromised rescue. The specialty-interest areas field has constructed and consensually validated these fragments. Experts can train FP specialists to appropriately use them.

The fourth area, "UT", represents unknown territory for the specialty-interest areas. A case falling into this classification is a situation that initially incurred because of error and/or an external pitfall. No whole or fragmented procedures or heuristics exist for dealing with this type of situation. This type of situation is outside of the field's zone of proximal development. Individualistic innovation (depicted as "I" in Figure 2) or referral is needed. If innovation fails, Brock (1979) explains that the medical facility should hold a mortality and morbidity (M and M) conference. If the FP specialist successfully innovates, the FP specialist should present the case in grand rounds (or the equivalent). If the case is well received, the FP specialist should write and submit the case for publication as a potential input for the field's ongoing construction and consensual validation process.

Resolving the Complex Dilemma

I discovered that the key to answering my main research question involves resolving the complex dilemma of specialty-interest areas in the FP field. The complex dilemma includes the autonomy/control dilemma and the safe/risk dilemma.

Way 1 and Way 2 do not resolve the complex dilemma. Each causes you to be hooked on the horns of the procedures/invention dilemma. Each leads FP specialists toward the autonomy horn when FP specialists try to figure out on their own how to recover from untoward events.

Way 3 resolves the complex dilemma by accepting:

- The risk horn as the syntonic while absorbing the safe horn as the dystonic without eliminating the safe horn
- The procedure horn as the syntonic and invention horn as the dystonic without eliminating the invention horn
- The control horn as the syntonic and autonomy horn as the dystonic without eliminating the autonomy horn

Way 3 shifts learners from having high levels of control (represented during cognitive apprenticeship phases one and two) to fading of that control (represented during cognitive apprenticeship phase three) to internalization (represented during cognitive apprenticeship phase 4). Internalization involves autonomy but with less autonomy than represented by the autonomy horn. Internalization is analogous to Thompson's (2993) bounded flexibility. In Figure 20, the cognitive-apprenticeship phases are represented by CA1, CA2, CA3, CA4, and CA5.

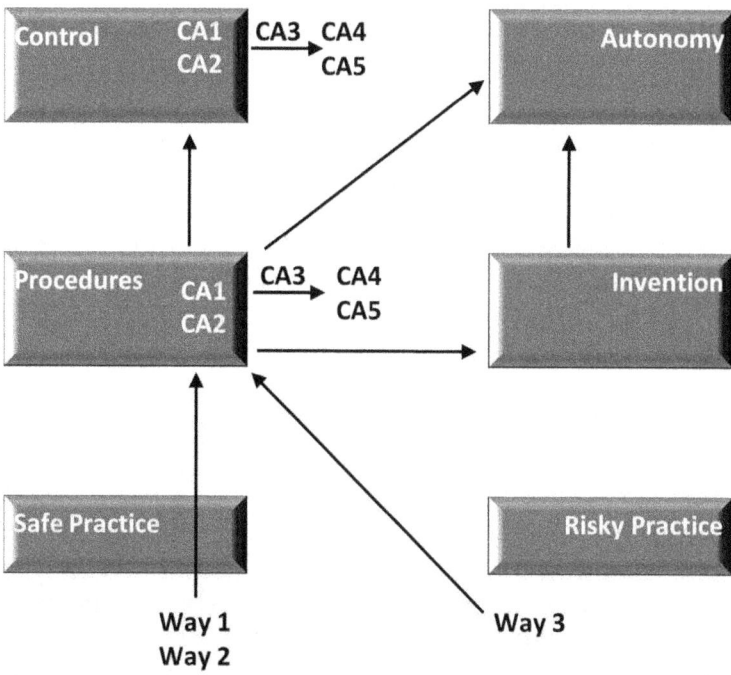

CA1 = First phase of cognitive apprenticeship (modeling with articulation)
CA2 = Second phase of cognitive apprenticeship (scaffolding and coaching)
CA3 = Third phase of cognitive apprenticeship (fading)
CA4 = Fourth phase of cognitive apprenticeship (internalization)
CA5 = Fifth phase of cognitive apprenticeship (generalization)

Figure 20. The Three Ways and the Complex Dilemma

The resolution of the complex dilemma with the primary consideration being whether the work is relatively safe or risky is consistent with Bandura's (1986) conditional knowledge for professional work as described in chapter 1.

When work is relatively safe, you can use any type of learning. When work is risky, only social-cognitive learning is appropriate for training.

Conditional Knowledge of the Types of Learning

Using Way 3 to learn the work proficiently as FP specialists who have developed specialty-interest areas and resolving the complex dilemma are supported by Bandura's (1986) contention that high-risk work should be learned through social-cognitive learning rather than trial-and-error learning. Cognitive apprenticeship operationalizes social-cognitive learning for high-risk work. Thus, you can operationalize Way 3 with cognitive apprenticeship.

Operationalizing Way 3

Cognitive Apprenticeship

Using cognitive apprenticeship to train FP specialists in high-risk fields operationalizes the social process and leads to bounded flexibility (cognitive apprenticeship phase four). Cognitive apprenticeship enables trainers to instructing practices that handle types of situations in ways that the profession considers as acceptable. In addition, cognitive apprenticeship clarifies the meaningfulness of learning. Ausubel et al. (1978) explains that learning becomes meaningful when the learning clarifies what need to do, want to do, and are doing in their practice of medicine or for helping them pass an examination such as a certificate of added qualification in specialty-interest areas.

In addition, learning must appropriate for the learners' zone of proximal development for the learning to be meaningful. Cognitive apprenticeship is a means to doing this.

BOGERD as Serving Cognitive Apprenticeship

Lippert et al. (1997) recommends the BOGERD technique for contracting meaningful supervised clinical training. I explain each phase below from the emerging viewpoint.

Background

In this phase, the trainer establishes the learners' zone of proximal development. The trainer determines the learners' previous experiences and expertise that can contribute to their understanding and abilities in applying the planned procedure.

Opportunity and goal

The trainer figures out how much and how quickly learners can be bootstrapped up their zone of proximal development. Resnick (1989) explains that bootstrapping avoids slow, trial-and-error learning. Bootstrapping situates the learning and by makes learning meaningful (Ausubal et al., 1978). Figuring out the amount of boot-strapping is based on the educational process of socialization and explanation.

Socialization

Socialization is carried out when the trainer models how to deal with a type of problem using an acceptable procedure (such as a gold standard that the profession has constructed and consensually validated) while avoiding unacceptable practices.

Explanation

Explanation is done when the trainer describes the underlying principles of the modeled procedure, any heuristics or tricks-of-the-trade that help make it work, and pitfalls that are likely to occur along with the proper associated risk management.

Evaluation

Offering feedback, both formative and summative promotes meaningfulness. The trainer's feedback reflects to the learners how well and how accurately they are progressing.

Rescue

Trainers model to learners the practice of risk management. This helps socialize them to handle lower-level risks and untoward events.

Deal

The learners must be shown how to define the roles of the trainer and trainee explicitly. The deal clarifies the role portrayed by each party, and it thereby eliminates the possibility for role confusion.

Bootstrapping and the Zone of Proximal Development

In handling untoward events, the zone of proximal development becomes a critical element in the socialization process and in determining how to manage constructive and destructive bugs. Figure 21 depicts the zone of proximal development for specialty-interest areas.

For trainers to instructed handling constructive bugs ethically and responsibly, trainers need to incorporate them when instructing procedures. Trainers must decide if learning how to manage a constructive bug is within the learners' zone of proximal development. If so, as depicted as "CB1" in Figure 21, then trainers explain when constructive bugs occur and model how to handle them. Thus, trainers present the conditional knowledge for handling constructive bugs. If the learners are not ready, as depicted as "DB1" in Figure 21, then trainers perceive the bugs to be destructive for learners, and trainers avoid putting learners in jeopardy by prematurely presenting the bugs and resolution to them. If presented prematurely, trainers would set the learners up for a guided shaming experience at best, and at worst, an untoward event. Thus, trainers must responsibly scaffold learners in their development. They need to bootstrap learners as effectively and efficiently as possible up through the learners' zone of proximal development to maximize competent practice.

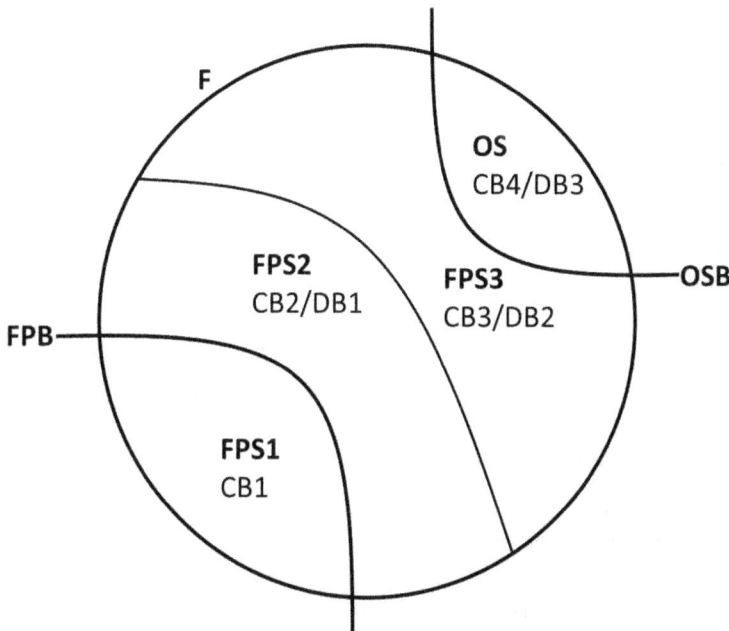

F   = Field's zone of proximal development of a specialty-interest
            area
FPB   = FP boundary
OSB   = Other specialty boundary
FPS1   = FP specialists getting started
FPS2   = FP specialists established
FPS3   = FP specialists well-established
OS   = Other type of specialist
CB1   = Constructive bugs for FP1
CB2/DB1 = Constructive bugs for FPS2 / destructive bugs for FPS1 field
CB3/DB2 = Constructive bugs for FPS3 / destructive bugs for FPS2 field
CB4/DB3 = Constructive bugs for OS / destructive bugs for FP field

Figure 21. Zone of Proximal Development for Specialty-Interest Areas

Specialty-interest areas have destructive bugs which FP specialists should avoid. Such bugs can only be handled by another type
of specialist, as depicted as "CB4/DB3" in Figure 21. Trainers need
to instruct learners how to find and avoid destructive bugs. As described in chapter 3, one well-established FP specialist found such
a situation. He said:

> In one case out of over a thousand vasecto-
> mies that I've done, I had to get help from a
> specialist. I called my urologist colleague

and said, "I have a patient who is bleeding
badly, and he is swelling to the size of a
grapefruit. I need your help." The urologist
came over, and we took the patient into surgery together. He found the artery causing
the problem and tied it.

Rather than trying to handle the complication alone, the FP specialist recognized that this was a destructive bug. He sought help from
another type of specialist trained to handle this type of bug (destructive for FP specialists and constructive for another type of specialist).

Summary of the Way 3

The BOGERD and cognitive-apprenticeship techniques operationalize the emerging viewpoint. The BOGERD technique con-
tracts with learners to instruct them the *need-to-do knowledgeably*
rather than the *need-to-know*. Through mastering that distinction,
learners can avoid the applicative fallacy. In addition, BOGERD
makes learning meaningful by first finding the learners' starting
point and then bootstrapping them within their zone of proximal development.

When actions are not risky, trainers can use any of the types of
learning. However, for situations that are risky, complex, ill-defined
or time-constrained, social learning is the only approach indicated.

The goal of the emerging viewpoint is to socialize learners to the
gold standards of the specialty-interest area. Encouraging learners
to invent their own gold standards is irresponsible and unethical.

The broad aim for new learners initially is to imitate or approximate the modeled gold standards with the trainer's assistance, and
then eventually perform those tasks unaided in ways that work for
them but still being within acceptable limits defined by the profession. I describe this broad aim as bounded flexibility.

Sigmoid Curve and Bounded Flexibility

In the construction of specialty-interest areas, the end goal is to
construct a bounded flexibility for handling various types of problems, situations, cases, and untoward events. While specialty-interest areas are emerging, it may be necessary but not desirable for

pioneers to innovate and invent (autonomous methods) for applying procedures, routines, protocol and risk management to the specialty-interest area's environment. This is depicted as "P" in Figure 22.

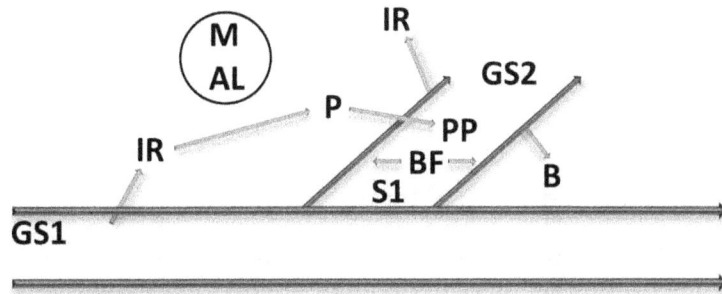

PP   = Proficient practices by FP specialists who have entered a specialty-interest area
S1   = Socialization of FP specialists to a specialty-interest area
GS1 = Gold standards of FP
GS2 = Gold standards of a specialty-interest area
BF   = Boundaries of the acceptable practice of gold standards
P   = Pioneers developing gold standards of an emerging specialty-interest area
B   = Practice inconsistent with the gold standards of a specialty-interest area
AL   = Adaptive leadership
M   = Models
I   = Innovation
R   = Research

Figure 22. Revised Sigmoid Curve Model for Specialty-Interest Areas

Pioneers of an emerging specialty-interest area may operate in isolation with no available models, but they can also recruit models from other disciplines to assist in the construction of the new gold standards. This is depicted as "M" in Figure 22. As the specialty-interest area practice becomes established, pioneers should discourage autonomous practice as the end-goal and help socialize new FP specialists developing the specialty-interest area by social learning theory. This is depicted as "S1" in Figure 22). Bootstrapping, cognitive apprenticeship, and BOGERD are means of socializing new FP specialists. These techniques require the end goal of having the FP specialists internalize the procedures and risk management into ways that work for them but remain within the boundaries as defined by that specialty-interest area's profession.

Handy (1994) and Heifietz (1996) describe professions as dynamic, and FP specialists must adapt as their environment and situations continually change. The need to engage in formal and informal networking is critical for adaption. While it is possible, but not desirable, to work in specialty-interest areas as an isolated (or detached) individual, working with a cadre of professionals encourages situated learning (Lave and Wenger, 1991) by socializing new FP specialists and enabling them to help one another improve and enhance the gold standards of the field.

Limitations of this Study

Before discussing implications for practice, consider these study limitations. The constant-comparative method of qualitative analysis is designed to construct and suggest theories. These theories have not been empirically tested using traditional quantitative approaches or non-experimental qualitative approaches.

While these theories apply to the small sampling of FP specialists at Carle Hospital, I cannot generalize these findings to the larger population of FP specialists who engage in specialty-interest areas. Moreover, I cannot generalize tentative implications to other specialty groups that engage in specialty-interest areas or sub-specializations.

Implications for Practice

Because the constant-comparative method of qualitative analysis is designed to generate and suggest (but not provisionally test) theories, categories, and hypotheses, experimental testing has not validated any of the following suggestions. Therefore, take caution for I make no attempt to generalize or prove suggested implications from my study.

Implications for FP Specialists Entering Specialty-Interest Areas

With few exceptions, specialty-interest areas are still emerging in the FP field, and therefore, FP specialists should take responsibility for their own development. Practitioners should recognize the importance of socialization to the currently known gold standards and avoid the applicative fallacy. Practitioners also should recognize how critical socialization is for ethical integration of specialty-interest areas in the FP specialists' clinical practice. All the following appear to be necessary for proficient practice:

- Seeking successful models
- Identifying and working with a cadre of professionals
- Being able to apply procedures
- Constructing proper risk management procedures with the help of other professionals

When new FP specialists pioneer a specialty-interest area, they should recruit assistance from specialists in relevant fields. For example, when a FP specialist wanted to construct therapeutic techniques in his clinical practice, he recruited a psychologist who advised him on applying counseling techniques. Recruitment of such experts, models, and adaptive leaders may be the key to constructing gold standards for new specialty-interest areas.

Implications for Continuing Medical Education, Residency Programs, and Medical Schools

Because medical practices are risky, have real time-constraints, are complex, and can be ill-defined, trainers need to use cognitive apprenticeship and the BOGERD techniques. Trainers can use both to construct meaningful supervised clinical education, and to help learners understand the proper ways to handle frequent problems and infrequent complications such as pitfalls and untoward events. Fundamental components of these techniques include risk management procedures for managing ill-defined problems and anomalies constitute. Trainers train learners the procedures along with training the pitfalls and risks. Because the procedures are interrelated with pitfalls and risks, pitfalls and risks should not be trained separately.

Implications for Adaptive Leadership

Adaptive leadership (Heifetz, 1996) involves bringing in FP specialists into specialty-interest areas. Adaptive leaders need to ensure that trainers socialize FP specialists using the emerging value. The following groups are positioned to offer adaptive leadership to FP specialists who are developing their specialty-interest areas:

- Departmental directors of attendings in family practice

- Specialists from other areas relevant to the specialty interest area (such as orthopaedics for sports medicine)
- FP specialists who are well established in a specialty-interest area
- Administrators

These professionals need to prevent FP specialists from trying to figure out the specialty-interest area (from the control or autonomy perspectives) individualistically.

Adaptive leaders need to turn pressure on and off to ensure that individuals and institutions address and work through the dilemma rather than allowing individuals to become trapped by the autonomy and control horns. Adaptive leaders need to help others realize that being hooked by the autonomy and control horns can lead to undesirable consequences in practice, patient care, and staff training.

Adaptive leaders need to connect FP specialists with relevant resources. This includes the models from related specialties and from the specialty-interest area who are using Way 3 and social-cognitive learning. Adaptive leaders need to introduce and socialize new FP specialists to existing networks of FP specialists who already function in the specialty-interest area. This can be done by:

- Electronic means
- Having them attend conferences and meetings where others present and interact within the specialty-interest areas

Networking with these FP specialists can help make explicit the issues of assimilation and accommodation within the specialty-interest area.

Suggestions for Future Research

As stated above and previously in chapter 2, the constant-comparative method of qualitative analysis doesn't test theories, categories, and hypotheses provisionally. Instead, this method is designed for suggesting and generating theories, hypotheses, conditions, consequences, dimensions, and processes. Future researchers may design studies to test these suggestions.

While I focused this study on FP specialists, researchers might consider examining how this applies for other specialists who sub-specialize (rather than enter specialty-interest areas). For example, a researcher could explore how general orthopaedic surgeons sub-specializing in ankle surgery and how they become socialized to that sub-specialty. Test questions could include the following:

- Do ankle sub-specialists have their own gold standards separate from general orthopaedics?
- What type(s) of learning best explain how orthopaedic surgeons sub-specialize?
- How do orthopaedic surgeons become socialized to sub-specialties?

Conclusion

My study focused on clinical practice of FP specialists who have developed specialty-interest areas without fully becoming another type of specialist. From my review of the literature and from interviews with FP specialists currently engaged in specialty-interest areas, I found and postulated a complex dilemma that FP specialists face when developing specialty-interest areas. To resolve this dilemma, I decided that trainers need to socialize FP specialists to:

- The gold standards of specialty-interest areas
- Risk management procedures for handling pitfalls and untoward events
- Avoid destructive bugs (when and how)

Because of the high-risk nature of clinical practice, trainers should primarily use social-cognitive learning. Other types of learning are useful in non-risky situations, but these are contraindicated for more complex, risky, ill-defined and time-consuming situations.

By using social-cognitive learning techniques such as cognitive apprenticeship and BOGERD, trainers can instruct in a situated and meaningful manner. Training this way expedites the learning process and bypasses those unethical training practices that promote trial-and-error learning to the detriment of the practice and its clients.

Glossary

accommodation: Professionals develop structures for interpreting new information. This also is known as restructuring.

assimilation: Professionals add new facts to their existing knowledge without changing the information-processing system itself. This also is known as accretion.

autonomous-learning technique: This technique is trial-and-error learning, where the learner invents the procedures.

Rather than receiving instructions from another person, the learner seeks to develop knowledge, attitudes, and skills independently. Although this may involve the reading of material, which is like reception learning, autonomous learning differs in that the learner chooses the necessary reading material and chooses the techniques for practicing or applying what is learned. West, Farmer, and Wolff (1991) caution using this approach in that the results may or may not produce desirable results for a given situation. Autonomous learning is primarily associated with humanistic philosophy and development.

Per Lave and Wenger (1991), professionals practice medicine instead of inventing it. They do not repeatedly discover procedures and subsequently retrieve what they discovered during clinical practice.

BOGERD technique: This technique, designed by Bulstrode and Hunt, is a supplementary process for cognitive apprenticeship. BOGERD contributes to cognitive apprenticeship and is a conceptual way of contracting meaningful supervised medical education.

This technique focuses on a clinical procedure and the appropriate time constraints.

The BOGERD technique has been adapted for use in cognitive apprenticeship (Lippert et al., 1997) to ensure that trainers meet the clinical learning needs and to ensure that responsible risk management takes place to protect patients, as much as possible, from untoward events.

Each letter stands for a phase of the sequential process:

1. Background
2. Opportunity
3. Goal
4. Evaluation
5. Rescue
6. Deal

Phases one and two need to occur before the other phases. Phases three, five, and six occur before cognitive apprenticeship starts. The fourth phase occurs throughout the training process. Before using BOGERD, the trainer selects a focal procedure that is part of the gold standards of the profession. Upon identifying this procedure, the trainer proceeds with the first phase of BOGERD.

bootstrapping: This is a metaphor for deliberately bypassing the slow and long part of the developmental learning curve in the professional clinical training of high-risk fields. Bootstrapping occurs using the cognitive-apprenticeship technique and involves avoiding trial-and-error learning.

Trainers determine how much and how quickly learners can be bootstrapped within their zone of proximal development.

bounded flexibility: This describes how FP specialists resolve the autonomy/control dilemma and is what I describe as the "emergent value." Bounded flexibility involves leveraging procedures that the FP profession has consensually validated while allowing some flexibility for autonomous action. FP specialists cannot follow procedures rigidly, but they follow them with a proper amount of flexibility to allow for autonomy and internalization. The field's consensually validated procedures bound the amount of autonomy.

cognitive-apprenticeship technique: This is designed to socialize learners to a field's gold standards (Collins, Brown, and Newman, 1929; Farmer, Buckmaster, and LeGrand, 1992; Brandt, Farmer, and Buckmaster, 1993). Instructors encourage learners to internalize and practice the gold standards in ways that work for them but within limits defined by the profession.

Cognitive apprenticeship can be used to instruct acceptable procedures defined by a profession while situating relevant principles and skills within a set of specified procedures. This is carried out by completing a sequence of phases described in appendix VII.

Cognitive apprenticeship is the only learning technique that situates learning to types of problems and explains how a field or profession handles those types of problems.

Constant-comparative method of qualitative analysis: Researchers use this technique to examine data and identify patterns that generate a theory or theories of how a social group functions. Marshall and Rossman (1989) describe this technique as an art that enables researchers to arrange categories to best help readers to understand the data. This involves coding data to help researchers find patterns that may not be clear to those within the social group or by outside observers.

constructive bugs: These types of bugs are pitfalls that can occur while using gold-standard procedures, and learners can handle them during cognitive apprenticeship. When trainers model handling microworlds or types of situations, they include instructions for handling constructive bugs.

Constructive bugs are within the learners' zone of proximal learning.

data display: This is the process of organizing information about data in the form of tables, matrices, and other visual presentations. The purpose is to visually present the categories studied. This process is a technique for displaying triangulation by comparing data from different sources.

data reduction: Researchers use this process to transform raw data into meaningful theories. One technique for doing this is the constant-comparative method.

Throughout the data reduction, researchers need to be aware that they easily could experience confirmation bias.

destructive bugs: These are pitfalls that learners are not able to handle on their own, nor can they learn to handle them responsibly at this point in their professional development.

Destructive bugs are outside the learners' zone of proximal learning.

family practice (FP): *Family practice* is a medical specialty that emphasizes "care of the individual, not as an isolated entity, but within the context of a family" (American Academy of Family Physicians, 1996). Family-practice departments offer broad-based services, which are "not limited by a patient's age, sex, involved organ system or disease entity" (American Academy of Family Physicians, 1996). FP medicine emphasizes comprehensive care, preventive medicine, and patient education.

family-practice specialist: FP specialists are medical doctors, doctors of osteopathy, nurse practitioners, and certified physician assistants who have been socialized to and now work within the field of family practice.

gold standard: In the singular form, *gold standard* refers to the range of practices that a profession has found to be acceptable. Family practice, for example, has a gold standard that creates boundaries within which FP specialists can ethically practice. Working outside this boundary is unacceptable, threatens quality of patient care, and may lead to litigation.

gold standards: In the plural form, *gold standards* refer to the procedures for dealing with types of medical cases for which a profession, specialty, or specialty-interest area has constructed and gained wide acceptance (i.e., consensually validated). For example, there are gold standards for setting fractures and gold standards for conducting general physical examinations. These gold standards operate within the gold standard of the profession, specialty, or specialty-interest area.

guided-inquiry technique: The philosophy of guided inquiry originates from the behaviorism and humanism learning orientations. Behavioral influences include setting goals of desired outcomes, breaking learning into parts, and using a stimulus/response technique in trial-and-error learning.

Guided inquiry encourages the invention and retrieval of medical procedures. Medicine is not invented but is practiced in a manner that has been constructed and consensually validated by the profession. However, phase four of guided inquiry encourages experimentation, which, even under the guidance of an attending, places patients at risk. In this phase, the instructor does not directly explain to the learner how the profession has determined how to deal with and handle such problems satisfactorily. As a result, phase four might lead to unintended and inappropriate learning of the procedures in which learners may mistakenly apply what was learned to handle other problems. Learners may not understand why such approximations can be harmful in different situations.

guided-shaming technique: This technique is a potential consequence of using guided inquiry for instructing medical procedures. Instructors encourage and allow learners to perform a procedure that the learners aren't developmentally prepared to handle. When learners fail in completing the procedure in the proper manner, instructors assume control of the situation, correct errors that were made by the learner, complete the procedure in the proper and satisfactory procedure, and often reprimand the learners for failing and causing potential or real harm to patients.

Possible motivation for using this technique includes a desire to humble learners and motivate learners to work harder in their development.

Per Resnick (1989), two negative consequences of guided shaming can occur:

1. Learners become less motivated to pursue their education, causing a downward spiral in learning.
2. If learners performed the procedure partially correctly and don't understand fully why their technique was inappropriate, learners could misapply their invented technique in the future. Resnick explains that instructors have difficulty trying to help

learners unlearn inappropriate techniques and misinformation.

Handy's inside-out doughnut: Handy's (1994) inside-out doughnut model graphically explains specialty-interest areas.
The conceptual model depicts a shape resembling a
doughnut with the hole on the outside and the dough in the
middle. In this model (depicted as figure 3), the core of the
doughnut holds the practice, in keeping with the gold
standards of family practice.

While many specialists learn to become an expert in the
core or the heart of the doughnut (Handy, 1994), some
choose to expand their core to include a specialty-interest
area. Per Handy, the core is not the whole doughnut. What
lie beyond the core are the degrees of freedom for adapting or shifting to a specialty-interest area.

horns of a dilemma: Dilemmas consist of two conflicting or opposing viewpoints, tendencies, perspectives, methods of
operation, or philosophical approaches (Petrie, 1991). Petrie metaphorically describes the diametric viewpoints as
horns of a dilemma.

The *horns of dilemma* are a bull metaphor. Accepting one
viewpoint over another is like being caught by one of a
bull's two horns: you'll experience negative consequences.

To resolve the dilemma, you need to go between the horns
by accepting both viewpoints. To do this, one viewpoint
needs to be *syntonic* and the other *dystonic.*

FP specialists must resolve three dilemmas. I describe
these as the *three-way interlocking dilemma.*

microworlds: This is a metaphor for types of situations that FP
specialists could encounter within their medical practice.
Trainers present types of medical situations and models of
how to handle them by applying appropriate procedures as
defined by the gold standards of FP, specialty-interest areas, or the specialty.

After learners become proficient in handling a set of microworlds, trainers introduce similar and more complex microworlds and models, showing how to handle them using
relevant gold-standard procedures.

proficient practice/proficiency: *Proficiency* is defined as the ability to handle a type of situation using an acceptable procedure that has been constructed and consensually validated by one's profession, specialty, or specialty-interest area for handling such situations while avoiding unacceptable practices (Lippert and Farmer, 1984).

quality assurance: *Quality assurance* involves dealing with common types of pitfalls that can occur within a procedure in which there are known ways for managing these pitfalls (Roberts, 1995).

reception-learning technique: In this approach, the learner merely receives the information. This occurs through reading, listening, or observing. The intent is for learners to understand and apply what is learned satisfactorily.

Unfortunately, learners often do not achieve this intent and experience what Farmer (1997) calls the *applicative fallacy*. The experience of observing a particular procedure being performed and reading documentations about a particular procedure is different from performing the actual procedure. Applicative fallacy relates to the post-hoc fallacy and the false-alternative fallacy.

Because of the potential risks to patient care, assuming that reception of information alone will instruct learners to apply procedures in a valid manner is unacceptable and irresponsible.

risk management: *Risk management* is a set of procedures for finding, evaluating, and correcting potential risks, which can cause harm to patients, professional staff, personnel, or property (Anderson, 1994).

The cornerstone of medical risk management is reflective medicine. Roberts (1995) explains that a FP specialist who uses reflective medicine "continuously recognizes medicine's ability to do harm, reflects on the patient's progress, and strives to keep the patient satisfied" (1678).

scaffolding: Brown and Palincsar (1989) describe *scaffolding* as an adjustable and temporary support. Expert trainers guide learners and provide support throughout the process. As learner skills increase, the amount of scaffolding decreases. If task difficulty increases, scaffolding increases as well. If learners experience unexpected challenges, trainers increase the scaffolding.

social-cognitive learning: This technique presupposes a triadic reciprocal model consisting of:

- Behavior
- Personal factors (cognition)
- Environmental events (social)

These elements interact with one another for explaining human function (Bandura, 1986).

Instructors should use the social-cognitive learning approach in high-risk professions in the form of *cognitive apprenticeship*. Cognitive apprenticeship can be supplemented with the concepts of *microworlds, constructive and destructive bugs,* and the *BOGERD technique.*

socialization: *Socialization* is an initiation process, part tacit and part explicit, into the elaborate and complicated environment of clinical practice. Socializing FP specialists to a specialty-interest area involves introducing and instructing specific knowledge and skills. Socialization involves acquiring the values and beliefs of the organization, including the following:

- Ethics
- Power structures
- Roles
- Standing traditions
- The jargon (Anderson, 1994)

Trainers model how to deal with a type of problem using an acceptable procedure, such as a gold standard, that the profession has constructed and consensually validated, in addition to models who avoid unacceptable practices.

Socratic-learning technique: Socratic learning (Segen, 1992) is an alternative teaching philosophy that instructs learners to invent ways of handling types of problems rather than having trainers socialize new learners to gold standards. Socratic learning involves having trainers ask questions designed to elicit contradictory inferences to eliminate inappropriate principles and procedures and to bring about the proper ways of handling certain types of situations. In doing so, instructors allow learners to invent their own methods for handling types of situations, which in turn encourages learners to use them to handle other types of situations when they are on their own.

Socratic learning encourages learners to develop individualistic innovations rather than practice consensually validated procedures by the profession.

Segen explains that the Socratic method is most effective in oral examinations and least effective for aiding in standardized examinations.

specialty-interest areas: *Specialty-interest areas* involve finding a niche in which to make a valuable and sometimes unique contribution. Specialty-interest areas can play an essential complementary role by bringing in what is needed from another field and/or by offering services more economically. FP specialists can develop a specialty-interest area within a department of family practice. They also can go into a specialty-interest area by finding a niche within another specialty area.

syntonic and dystonic: I use these terms to describe how FP specialists resolve dilemmas. To resolve the dilemmas, FP specialists must accept both choices rather than just one. One choice becomes the primary approach, which is the *syntonic.* The other choice is the secondary approach, which is the *dystonic.*

For example, with the control/autonomy dilemma, FP specialists need to work primarily from a control perspective, the *syntonic,* but still need to be autonomous, the *dystonic,* in certain situations. Autonomy is practiced within *bounded flexibility.* FP specialists would be irresponsible if they followed procedures rigidly or if they only behaved autonomously without accepting the constraints of the procedures.

three-way interlocking dilemma: When expanding from family
medicine to specialty-interest areas, FP specialists must
resolve a complex dilemma. The dilemma consists of three
separate but interrelated dilemmas. The three-way interlocking dilemmas are as follows:

- Control vs. autonomy
- Procedure vs. invention
- Safe practice vs. risky practice

These dilemmas are complexly interrelated because FP
specialists can shift how they become entangled in the interlocking dilemma in different ways, depending on the circumstances of the situation. Different environmental factors, personal factors, and behavioral factors may influence
how FP specialists become caught in the dilemma.

To mitigate confusion and problematic thinking, FP specialists need to resolve this complex dilemma.

zone of proximal development: In the traditional sense, the
zone of proximal development, or ZPD, is the range of
tasks or procedures that can be learned with instruction.
Outside the ZPD are tasks or procedures that learners
cannot perform even with instruction at a particular time.

For example, Sam is learning geometry. He is within his
ZPD if he has learned algebra already. Advanced calculus
would be outside of Sam's ZPD because has hasn't
learned enough mathematics yet.

In the context of this research, FP specialists have already
completed their formal training in family medicine. Learning
a specialty-interest area is within FP specialists' ZPD. For
example, Heather, a FP specialist, could learn the specialty-interest area of sports medicine. However, learning
another specialty such as orthopaedic surgery is outside
her ZPD. An artificial disc replacement procedure (arthro-
plasty) is a specific example of a procedure that Heather
wouldn't perform when learning sports-medicine procedures.

Cover Letter for Survey

February 11, 1998

[family-practice specialist's Name]
[Department Name]
[City location]

Subject: Request for dissertation participants from Family Practice

Dear **[Name]**,

I am writing to ask you to participate in my doctoral thesis. The focus of my study is on how family-practice specialists develop specialty interest areas. If you have currently integrated a specialty interest area into your clinical practice, please complete the enclosed survey and use the attached envelope and routing slip.

The sole purpose of the enclosed survey is for you to nominate yourself for an interview. If you volunteer for an interview, I will schedule the interview at your site and at your convenience.

Thank you again for your time and consideration,

Gary DePaul, M.Ed.
Doctoral Candidate

Enclosures: Letter of Consent (please return with survey)
              Letter of Consent (for your records)
              Survey
              Return Envelope
              Return address for Carle mail system

Letter of Consent

You are invited to participate in a research project, which focuses on how family-practice specialists develop specialty interest areas. This study will be conducted by Gary DePaul as partial fulfillment of his Doctorate of Philosophy in continuing Education at the University of Illinois. The project chair is Dr. James A. Farmer, Professor, Department of Educational Organization and Leadership.

In this study, participants will be asked to complete a one-page survey to help identify specialty interest areas within family practice. Based on survey results, you may be asked to participate in a one-hour individual interview or a one-hour focus group. In these interviews and focus groups, which will be audiotaped, participants will be asked to discuss their experiences in developing specialty interest areas within family practice. The audiotapes and all information collected from this study will be kept anonymous and confidential. Your participation in this study is completely voluntary, and you are free to withdraw at any time and for any reason without penalty. There are no risks or discomforts expected to occur from participating in the survey or from the interviews. You may, at any point, decline to answer specific questions on the survey or in the interview or focus group sessions.

Participants will receive an executive summary of the results upon completion of this project.

I understand that in the event of physical injury resulting from this research, there is no compensation available for such injury and that any necessary medical care required will be handled in the same way as my usual medical care.

I understand that a record of my participation in the study will be kept in confidential form and that confidentiality is carefully guarded. During their required reviews, representatives of the Food and Drug Administration (FDA) have access to medical records which contain my identity; however, no information by which I can be identified will be released or published.

If I wish to speak to a party not associated with this research and to whom I may address complaints about this study as well as concerns about my rights as a participant, I may contact the Department of Medical Research at 217/383-3036.

If you have any questions about this research project that you wish to direct to the researcher, please call Gary DePaul at 217/344-8757 or Dr. James Farmer at 217/333-2155.

I have read and understand the above information and voluntarily agree to participate in the research project described above. I have been offered a copy of this consent form.

_____
Signature and Date of Participant

Carle
I.R.B.
approved
consent form
Valid until:
10/15/98

_____
Signature of Witness

_____
Signature of the Principal Investigator

Survey Questionnaire

Introduction
This research project is an exploratory study designed to identify family practice specialists (i.e., medical doctors, physician assistants, and nurse practitioners) who have gone into a specialty-interest area but who have not become another type of specialists.

Examples
A family-practice physician who has a strong interest in muscular skeletal illnesses and injuries and who has integrated a considerable amount of muscular skeletal work within his practice is an example of a specialty-interest area in orthopaedics without becoming an orthopaedic surgeon.

A family-practice nurse practitioner who works in the Cardiology Department.

Instructions
If you have a specialty-interest area, please answer all questions. If you do not have a specialty-interest area, please ignore this survey questionnaire.

1. Do you have a specialty-interest area
within your current practice?   Yes   No

If so, in what? _____

2. To what extent have you developed this specialty-interest area
    (without becoming another type of specialist)? Please respond
    by marking on the line:

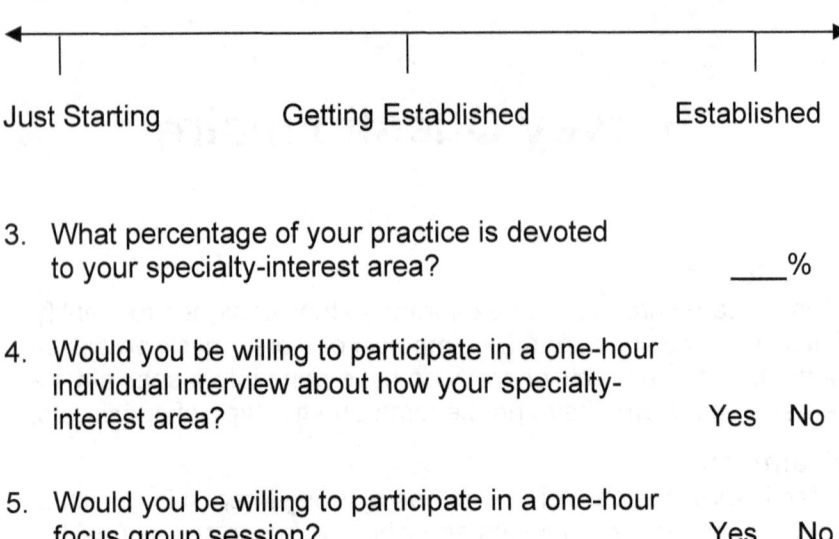

Just Starting   Getting Established   Established

3. What percentage of your practice is devoted
    to your specialty-interest area?   ____%

4. Would you be willing to participate in a one-hour
    individual interview about how your specialty-
    interest area?   Yes   No

5. Would you be willing to participate in a one-hour
    focus group session?   Yes   No

Initial Questions for One-On-One Interviews

1. What Type of Work Do You Do?

2. How Experienced Are You in Your Specialty-Interest Area?

3. Is the Clinical Practice of Your Specialty-Interest Area Considered to be Risky?

4. How Did You Learn To Manage Untoward Events Associated with Doing Procedures in Your Specialty-Interest Area?

5. What Formal and Informal Support Networks Are Available in Your Specialty-Interest Area?

6. How Did You Learn Your Specialty-Interest Area?

7. How Do You Teach Others Your Specialty-Interest Area? If You Don't Teach it, How Would You Teach This Area to Another Specialist?

8. How Has Family Practice Contributed To Your Specialty-Interest Area?

9. How Has Specialty-Interest Areas Contributed To Family Practice?

Revised Questions for One-On-One Interviews

1. What Type of Work Do You Do?

2. How Experienced Are You in Your Specialty-Interest Area?

3. If errors occur within a procedure and/or if unforeseen events complicate a procedure, can untoward events occur?

4. How Did You Learn To Manage Untoward Events Associated with Doing Procedures in Your Specialty-Interest Area?

5. What Formal and Informal Support Networks Are Available in Your Specialty-Interest Area?

6. How Did You Learn Your Specialty-Interest Area?

7. How Do You Teach Others Your Specialty-Interest Area? If You Don't Teach it, How Would You Teach This Area to Another Specialist?

8. How Has Family Practice Contributed To Your Specialty-Interest Area?

9. How Has Specialty-Interest Areas Contributed To Family Practice?

Roles of the Cognitive Apprenticeship Model

Phase	Role of learners	Role of Trainer
1	Observes both the overall procedure as well as the competencies. Begins to understand the schema or mental model of what the procedure looks like in actual practice	Models an acceptable procedure that has been constructed and consensually validated by the field for which the learners want to perform satisfactorily. States aloud the essence of the procedure including the underlying principles, pitfalls, and heuristics or tricks-of-the-trade.
2	In a controlled environment, approximate doing the actual procedure while articulating its essence (i.e., the principles, pitfalls, and heuristics or tricks-of-the-trade). Use self-monitoring and self-correction. Reflect on the model's performance	Provides coaching and support as needed. The trainer "checks out" the learners to make sure that they are following the procedures correctly
3	Continue to approximate the procedure. Work individually or with others.	Decreases the amount of coaching and scaffolding. Provides support as needed

Phase	Role of learners	Role of Trainer
4	Practice applying and performing the procedure in the actual cases but only within the range of the profession's acceptable practice and standards	Provides help only when requested
5	Discuss the generalizability of what was learned from the procedure	Explains the generalizability to other procedures by emphasizing commonalties and not just differences

Adapted from Brandt et al. (1993), Farmer et al. (1992), and Collins et al. (1989).

References

Arnold, D.J. (1970). Dimensional sampling: An approach for studying a small number of cases. *The American Sociologist*, <u>23</u>, 87-93.

American Academy of Family Physicians. (1996, December 13). *What they won't tell you about family practice....* Retrieved March 24, 1998 from the World Wide Web: http://www.aafp.org/family/student/spchoice.html

Anderson, K. N. (Ed.). (1994). *Mosby's medical, nursing, and allied health dictionary* (4th ed.). St. Louis: Mosby.

Ausubal, D. P., Novak, J. D., Hanesian, H. (1978). *Educational psychology: A cognitive view* (2nd Ed.). New York: Holt, Rinehart, and Winston.

Bandura, A. (1986). Social foundations of thought and action: A social cognitive theory. Englewood Cliffs, NJ: Prentice Hall.

Biklen, S.K., and Bodan, R. C. (1986). On your own with naturalistic evaluation. *New Dimensions for Program Evaluation, 30*, 93-101.

Bosk, C. L. (1979). *Forgive and remember: Managing medical failure*. Chicago: The University of Chicago Press.

Brandt, B. L., Farmer, J. A, Jr., and Buckmaster, A. (1993). Cognitive apprenticeship approach to helping adults learn. *New directions for adult and continuing education, 59*, 69-78.

Brown, A. L., and Palincsar, A.S. (1989). Guided, Cooperative Learning and Individual Knowledge Acqusition. *Knowing, learning, and instruction: Essays in honor of Robert Glaser* (pp.393-451). (L.B. Resnick, Ed). Hillsdale, New Jersey: Lawrence Erlbaum Associates.

Burton, R. R., Brown, J. S., and Fisher, G. (1984). Skiing as a model of instruction. In B. Rogoff and J. Lave (Eds.), *Everyday cognition: Its development in social context* (pp. 139-150). Cambridge, MA: Harvard University Press.

Candy, P. (1991). Self-direction for lifelong learning: A comprehensive guide to theory and practice. San Francisco: Josey-Bass.

Collins, A., Brown, J. S., and Newman, S. E. (1989). Cognitive apprenticeship: Teaching the craft of reading, writing, and mathematics. In Resnick, L. B. (Ed.), *Cognition and instruction: Issues and agendas.* Hillsdale, NJ: Lawrence Erlbaum Associates.

Dexter, L. A. (1970). *Elite and specialized interviewing.* Evanston: Northwestern University Press.

The directory of family practice residency programs. (1996). Chicago: American Academy of Family Practice.

Farmer, J. A., Jr. (1997). *New paradigm for orthopaedic education.* Unpublished manuscript.

Farmer, J. A., Jr., Buckmaster, A., and LeGrand, B. (1992). Cognitive apprenticeship: Implications for continuing professional education. *New directions for adult and continuing education, 55,* 41-50.

Farmer, J. A., Jr., Gilbert, L., Murray, S., Snellen., J., Bragg, D., Deschler., D., and Paprock, K. (1991). *Customer Satisfaction Assessment System* (Task Order 91-1). Champaign: University of Illinois, Office for the Study of Continuing Education, Training, and Development.

Feinstein, R. E., and Carey, L. (1995). Crisis intervention in office practice. In R. E. Rakel (Ed.), *Textbook for Family Practice* (5th ed.) (pp. 1502-1509). Philadelphia: W B Saunders Company.

Gagne, R. M. (1985). *The conditions of learning* (4th ed.). NY: Holt, Rinehart and Winston.

Glaser, B. G., and Strauss, A. L. (1973). *The discovery of grounded theory: Strategies for qualitative research.* Chicago: Aldine Publication Company.

Graduate medical education directory (1997-1998). Dover, DE: American medical Association.

Green, K. A. (1997). *Customer satisfaction with the Executive Veterinary Certificate Program in Swine Health Management.* Unpublished doctoral dissertation, University of Illinois, Urbana-Champaign.

Handy, C. (1994). *The age of paradox.* Boston: Harvard Business School Press.

Heifetz, R. A. (1994). *Leadership without easy answers.* Cambridge, MA: The Belknap Press of Harvard University Press.

Holleman, W. L., and Brody, B. A. (1995). Ethics in family practice. In R. E. Rakel (Ed.), *Textbook for Family Practice* (5th ed.) (pp. 153-162). Philadelphia: W B Saunders Company.

Jonassen, Hannum, and Tessmer (1989). *Handbook of task analysis procedures.* New York: Praeger Publishers.

Kekes, J. (1980). *The nature of philosophy.* Totowa, NJ: Rowman and Littlefield.

Kimmel D. C. (1980). *Adulthood and aging.* New York: John Wiley and Sons.

Krathwohl, D. R. (1993). Methods of Educational and social science research: An integrated approach. White Plains, NY: Longman.

Kuhn, T. S. (1970). *The structure of scientific revolutions, second edition.* Chicago: The University of Chicago Press.

Landra, L. N. (1984). The algo-heuristic theory of performance, learning, and instruction: Subject, problems, and instruction. *Contemporary Education Psychology, 9,* 235-245.

Lave, J. and Wenger E., (1991). *Situated learning: Legitimate peripheral participation.* New York: Cambridge University Press.

Lippert, F. G. (1997). Sample problem of use of heuristic strategies. In F. G. Lippert, J. F. Sarwark, J. J. Murnaghan, and J. A. Farmer, *Handbook for orthopaedic educators* (19th ed.), (pp. 129-122). Chicago: American Academy of Orthopaedic Surgeons.

Lippert, G., and Farmer, J. (1984). *Psychomotor skills in ortho-paedic surgery.* Baltimore: Williams and Wilkins.

Lippert, F. G., Farmer, J. A., Murnaghan, J. J., and Sarwark, J. F. (1997). *Handbook for orthopaedic educators* (19th ed.). Chicago: American Academy of Orthopaedic Surgeons.

Lincoln, Y. S., and Guba, E. G. (1985). *Naturalistic inquiry.* Beverly Hills, CA: Sage Publication.

Marshall, C., Rossman, G. B. (1989). *Designing qualitative research.* Newbury Park, CA: SAGE Publications, Inc.

Merriam, S. B. (1988). Case study research in education: A qualitative approach. San Francisco: Jossey-Bass.

Merton, R. K. (1968). *Social theory and social structure.* New York: The Free Press.

Mintzberg, H. (1994). The rise and fall of strategic planning: Reconceiving roles for planning, plans, planners. New York: The Free Press.

Petry, J., A. (1991). A case study in adult education: Strategies to teach computer concepts and procedures. University of Illinois at Urbana-Champaign.

Rakel, R. E. (1995). The family physician. In R. E. Rakel (Ed.), *Textbook for Family Practice* (5th ed.) (pp. 3-19). Philadelphia: W B Saunders Company.

Resnick, LB. (1989). Introduction. *Knowing, learning, and instruction: Essays in honor of Robert Glaser* (pp. 1-24). (L.B. Resnick, Ed). Hillsdale, New Jersey: Lawrence Erlbaum Associates.

Roberts, R. G. (1995). Malpractice and risk management. In R. E. Rakel (Ed.), *Textbook for Family Practice* (5th ed.) (pp. 1673-1683). Philadelphia: W B Saunders Company.

Rosenshine, B., and Meister, C. (1992). The use of scaffolds for teaching higher-level cognitive strategies. *Educational Leadership, 49,* pp. 26-33.

Rumelhart, D. E., and Norman, D. A. (1978). Accretion, tuning, and restructuring: Three types of learning. In J. Cotton, and R. L. Klatzky (Eds.), *Semantic factors in cognition* (pp. 37-60). NY: John Wiley and Sons.

Schumacher and McMillan (1993). *Research in education: A*

conceptual introduction (Third Ed.). New York: Harper Collins College Publishers.

Segen, J. C. (Ed.). (1992). *The dictionary of modern medicine.* Park Ridge, NJ: The Parthenon Publishing Group.

Senge, P. M., Kleiner, A., Roberts, C., Ross, R. B., Smith, B. J., (1994). *The fifth discipline fieldbook: Strategies and tools for building a learning organization.* New York: Doubleday.

Sommers, C. D. (1997). *Instruction in a nuclear reactor control room simulator.* Unpublished doctoral dissertation, University of Illinois, Urbana-Champaign.

The directory of family practice residency programs (1996). American Academy of Family Physicians.

Thompson, S.C. (1993). "Natural occurring perceptions of control: A model of bounded flexibility," In Weary, G., Gleicher, F., and Marsh, K. (eds.), *Control motivation and social cognition,* (pp. 74-93).

West, C. K., Farmer, J. A., and Wolff, P. M. (1991). *Instructional design: Implications from cognitive science.* Englewood Cliffs, NJ: Prentice Hall.

Yin, R. K. (1989). *Case study research: Design and methods.* Newbury Park, CA: Sage Publications.

Vygotsky, L. S. (1992). *Thought and language.* Cambridge, MA: The MIT Press.

Vygotsky, L. S. (1978). *Mind in society: The development of higher psychological processes.* (M. Cole, V. John-Steiner, S. Scribner, and E. Souberman, Eds.). Cambridge, MA: Harvard University Press.

Zelditch, M. (1962). Some methodological problems of field studies. *American Journal of Sociology, 67,* 566-576.

Acknowledgements from the First Edition

I would like to acknowledge the Carle Foundation Hospital and Carle Clinic Association for allowing me to conduct this study with their family-practice specialists.

Thanks to the dissertation committee members, Terry Hatch, Thomas McGreal, and Paul Thurston, for their feedback, support and contributions. Without their insights, aspects of this study would not have been realized. I particularly thank Terry Hatch for helping me navigate and understand the Carle system. Along with the committee, I thank Barbara Huffman and Stanley Levy for mentoring me, support, and feedback.

Thanks to the staffs of the Office of Educational Technology and Department of Educational Organization and Leadership for giving technical resources. Specifically, I thank Cathy Thurston, Linda Alexander, Shirley Fryer, and Diana Whitt.

Special thanks to Lulu Kurman for editing this manuscript. Along with Lulu, thanks to Sara Sasse for her editing, technical support, and suggestions.

One of the lessons learned from this process is that research is not performed in isolation. I thank my colleagues who are working on this line of inquiry. Specific members include Mavis Green, Steve Murray, Kathy Wehrmann, Michael Higgins, and Nancy Barrett. I especially thank Brent Williams, a colleague who is a voice of reason and friend.

I thank my parents for believing in me, for believing that I would finish, but mostly for giving unconditional love and support.

Lastly, I thank James Farmer, Jr. who has been my advisor and mentor. No one has influenced my professional outlook as much as Jim. Regardless of where my career takes me, the knowledge, skills, and values that I learned from Jim will carry over to strengthen my success. Thank you, Jim.

ABOUT THE AUTHOR

"I help professionals become more
effective at helping others develop."

Gary is an author, speaker, and leadership advisor with Gary De-
Paul Leadership Consulting. With more than 20 years of practitioner and academic experience in performance improvement, talent development, and knowledge management, Gary helps professionals become more effective at helping others develop.

Practitioner Experience

Gary has served executives and teams in both international and
national organizations including:

- Lowe's Companies Inc.
- Ceridian Benefits Services
- Fidelity Information Services
- Johnson Controls Inc.
- Arthur Andersen LLP

He has held formal roles including senior manager of training and
knowledge management, senior instructional designer, performance-improvement director, and workforce readiness manager.

Through these roles, he's develop expertise in project-manage-
ment methodology, human performance improvement, knowledge
management, training and talent development, and leadership.

Academic and Credential Experiences

At the University of Illinois at Urbana-Champaign, Gary completed his PhD and EdM through the Department of Educational Organization and Leadership.

He completed his bachelor's degree in history and philosophy from the University of Alabama at Birmingham.

The International Society for Performance Improvement designated him a certified performance technologist.

Speaking Experience

Gary has conducted workshops and sessions for companies and at international and national conferences. He has guest lectured at Notre Dame's Mendoza College of Business and at the University of North Carolina at Charlotte's Belk College of Business. He has presented to chambers of commerce as well as associations or their affiliated chapters including:

- International Society for Performance Improvement
- Association for Talent Development
- Society for Human Resource Management
- International Coach Federation
- Society for Technical Communication
- Project Management Institute

Recent presentations include:

- What Everyone Should Know about Leadership
- How Leadership Is Radically Changing: Implications for Talent Development
- The Wrong Way and Right Way to Develop Your Leadership
- Leadership Development: What Every Learning and Development Professional Should Know

Publication Experience

Gary has written performance-improvement articles for PerformanceXpress.com and Performance Improvement Journal.

In *The Trainer's Portable Mentor*, he coauthored an article with Donald Kirkey on formative evaluation.

While in graduate school at the University of Illinois at Urbana-Champaign, Gary was one of many coauthors of two evaluation articles published under the mentorship of Robert Stake.

Contact Information

If you are interested in contacting Gary about speaking or consulting, he can be reached through his website or by email:

- https://www.garyadepaul.com
- gary@garyadepaul.com

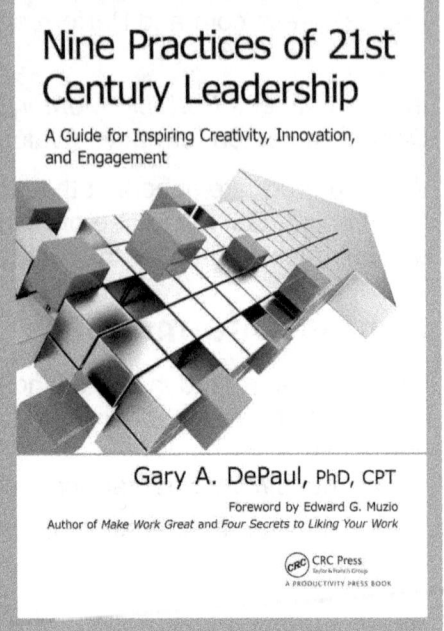
"Gary has saved anyone with an interest in the topic of leadership a tremendous amount of legwork and created an incredible resource for leadership growth. Most importantly, the rich assortment of examples, practices, and recommended actions provided are a tremendous asset to our development and growth as leaders. A note of caution: be prepared to see yourself and your own leadership assumptions and practices challenged (in a good way)."

Rick Rummler, President of The Rummler Group
Co-author of *White Space Revisited: Creating Value through Process*

"Gary DePaul's comprehensive *Nine Practices of 21st Century Leadership* makes sense of the vast sea of leadership books. Written with both managers and scholars in mind, DePaul's study situates--and demystifies--the language of leadership in systems thinking. In 15 well-organized and lucidly written chapters, the author builds a series of metaphors to explain the practices of expert managers--analyzing, detecting, guiding, nurturing and more. This book will change your thinking about leadership."

Edwin Battistella, Ph.D.
Author of *Sorry about That: The Language of Public Apology*

Forthcoming Books by Gary A. DePaul

Available in 2017

Crack the Leadership Development Codes
Stories of How Organizations Train Executives and Employees to Lead

Available in Late 2017 or Early 2018

Culture Growth
Expand Your Leadership Mindset, Transform Your Culture!

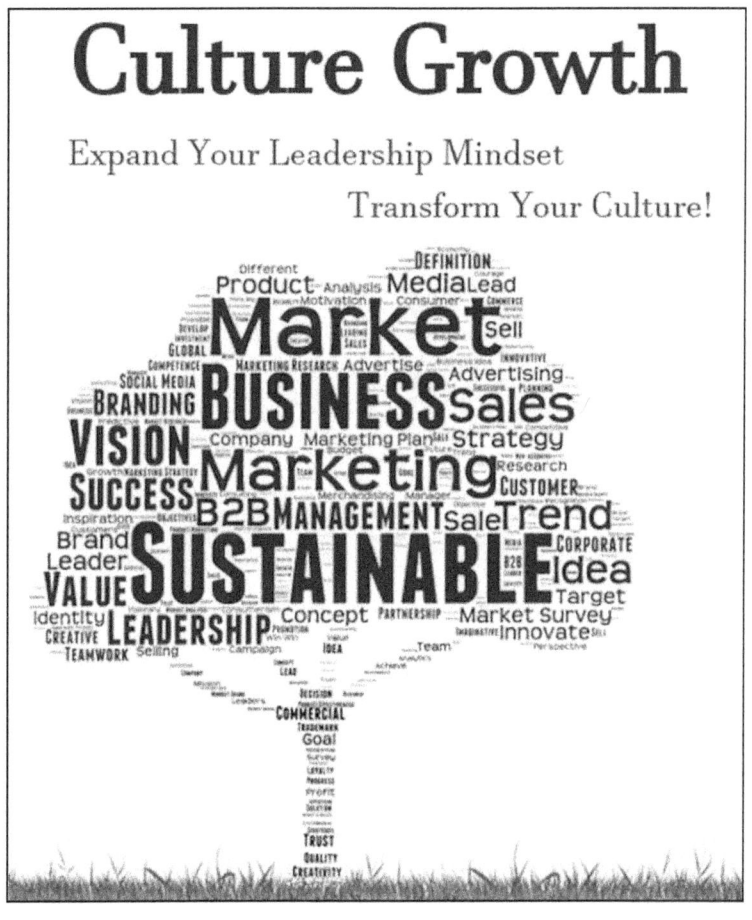